FRCR Part 1 Anatomy Mock Examinations

D1477319

FRCR Part 1 Anatomy
Mock Examinations

Aidan Shaw
Radiology Specialist Registrar,
Guy's and St Thomas' Hospitals, London

Benjamin Smith
Radiology Specialist Registrar,
Guy's and St Thomas' Hospitals, London

David C. Howlett
Radiology Consultant, Eastbourne District General Hospital,
Eastbourne, Reader in Imaging and Electronic Learning,
Brighton and Sussex Medical School and Royal College
of Radiologists Fellowship Examiner in Anatomy

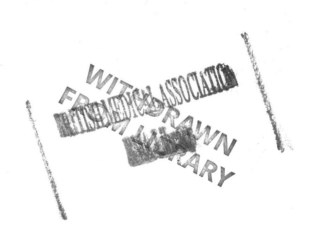

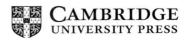
CAMBRIDGE
UNIVERSITY PRESS

CAMBRIDGE UNIVERSITY PRESS
Cambridge, New York, Melbourne, Madrid, Cape Town,
Singapore, São Paulo, Delhi, Tokyo, Mexico City

Cambridge University Press
The Edinburgh Building, Cambridge CB2 8RU, UK

Published in the United States of America by
Cambridge University Press, New York

www.cambridge.org
Information on this title: www.cambridge.org/9781107648647

First published 2011

Printed in the United Kingdom at the University Press, Cambridge

A catalogue record for this publication is available from the British Library

Library of Congress Cataloguing in Publication data
Shaw, Aidan.
  FRCR part 1 anatomy mock examinations / Aidan Shaw, Benjamin Smith,
  David C. Howlett.
    p. ; cm.
  ISBN 978-1-107-64864-7 (pbk.)
  1. Human anatomy – Great Britian – Examinations, questions, etc.
  2. Anatomy – Great Britian – Examinations, questions, etc.   I. Smith, Benjamin, 1979–
  II. Howlett, David C.   III. Royal College of Radiologists (Great Britain)   IV. Title.
  [DNLM: 1. Anatomy – Great Britain – Examination Questions.   2. Radiology –
  Great Britain – Examination Questions. QS 18.2]
  QM32.S33   2011
  612.0076–dc23   2011018897

ISBN 978-1-107-64864-7 Paperback

*Dedicated with love and gratitude to my mother, father and Juliette.
And to Jon Lund, to whom I shall always remain indebted. (AS)*

*To my dear wife Maeve, for all her love and support, and
to my parents, who have always been there for me. (BS)*

*To my dear wife, Joanna, and the children, Tom, Ella,
Robert and Miles, and also for Christopher. (DH)*

*To my wife, Siobhan, and four children, Emily,
Hugh, Annabel and Miles. (NT)*

Nicholas Taylor

Nicholas Taylor is a medical photographer with over thirty years of experience. He trained at Guy's Hospital before taking up posts at hospitals on the south coast, and has been the Senior Medical Photographer at Eastbourne District General Hospital for the last twenty years. He is a member of the Institute of Medical Illustrators and a registered medical illustration practitioner.

His role within the department has enabled him to contribute images and illustrations to numerous articles, journals and medical textbooks, as well as local history books of the Eastbourne area.

Recently, he has been responsible for the preparation of images for hundreds of medical cases for the e-learning element of undergraduate medical teaching on behalf of the Brighton and Sussex Medical School.

His expertise means that the Royal College of Radiologists has entrusted him with preparing the images for the FRCR Part 1 exams, and thus the standard of images used within this book equates very closely with those that will be found in the exams.

We, the authors, would like to pay tribute and give our immense thanks and gratitude to Nicholas Taylor for all his hard work on this book, from the front cover to the back page.

Contents

Foreword

Examinations may not be the most popular aspect of medical training but they are an essential part of our education system and make an important contribution to the very high standard of medicine in the United Kingdom. Structured testing is an objective and effective method of testing knowledge. This is especially true in the field of radiology, as it is possible to combine questions with images, thus bringing this form of testing closer to the reality of everyday life than is possible in many other medical specialities. Dr Aidan Shaw, Dr Benjamin Smith and Dr David Howlett have produced an outstanding book, which combines searching questions, testing important aspects of radiological anatomy, with excellent images that clearly demonstrate the findings. The questions are clear, succinct and readable and the quality of the images is superb. I believe that this book will prove very popular with radiologists preparing for examinations and will make revision (almost) a pleasure!

Andy Adam

Professor Andy Adam,
Professor of Interventional Radiology

Introduction

In 2010 the Royal College of Radiologists reintroduced the anatomy component of the FRCR Part 1 examination. The primary aim of this book is to provide trainee radiologists with a focused and invaluable revision aid when preparing for this exam. Its utility is not just limited to radiologists, however, and other groups such as radiographers and medical students will also find the detailed images and descriptions helpful to their studies. This book was written to be complementary to existing formal anatomy texts, and is intended to be used in conjunction with them.

The ten mock examinations within this book have been designed to closely conform with the new syllabus set out by the RCR. Each exam is laid out and structured in the same way as the actual papers, ensuring that readers will gain familiarity with both the content and the style of the examination. By the end of the book, readers will have encountered every imaging modality and the majority of cases covered in the exam itself. The answer sections include detailed explanations of the relevant anatomy, along with helpful learning tips and clinical applications.

The anatomy syllabus is available on the college website and should be studied closely. It is broadly divided into four categories: head and neck; thorax; abdomen and pelvis; and musculoskeletal system. Candidates can expect the examination to have roughly equal proportions from each category in the examination. It is specified in the 2010 syllabus that paediatric imaging of all ages will be included. Nuclear medicine, including positron emission tomography, is specifically excluded from the anatomy curriculum. All other major imaging modalities will be used in the exam, including radiographs, fluoroscopy, CT, MRI and ultrasound.

The new FRCR Part 1 anatomy examination is 75 minutes long and consists of 20 radiological images with five questions on each. Candidates will view the images on Apple Mac Mini workstations equipped with 19" monitors and running Osirix image-viewing software. Answers will be hand-written and are to be recorded in the provided question booklet.

To gain maximum marks for each question, the candidate must correctly identify the labelled structure and, if applicable, state which side the structure is on. For instance, answering 'kidney' might earn half of the marks, whereas answering 'right kidney' would earn the maximum credit. If the candidate gives the wrong side then no marks are awarded, so guessing is not recommended. If the labelled structure is a vertebra or nerve root, be sure to include the level in the answer if possible. Where the side is already provided in the question it is not necessary to repeat this in the answer. The candidate must ensure that the answer is legible and spelt correctly.

The majority of questions in the exam simply ask the candidate to name the labelled anatomical structure. There are some questions that go beyond this and further test anatomical knowledge. Examples of these include, 'What anatomical variant is present on the image?' and, 'What attaches to the labelled structure?' It is therefore extremely important to read each question carefully to ensure an appropriate answer is given.

So how can the reader best prepare for the new FRCR Part 1 anatomy exam? As always, it is advisable to start preparing well in advance and avoid last minute cramming in the final few days. It is worth using a variety of revision aids, including established anatomy textbooks, radiological atlases and practice papers. The mock exams in this book will be invaluable preparation, and we recommend that at some point the reader should attempt them under exam conditions to get a feel of the pace required. Perhaps the best advice we can offer is: read each question carefully and always, always remember to name the side.

It is possible that the exam format may change over the coming years, although the basic concept of an annotated image and five labels is likely to be retained and, as such, this book will act as a valuable revision aid regardless of how questions are structured.

Examination 1: Questions

Question 1.1

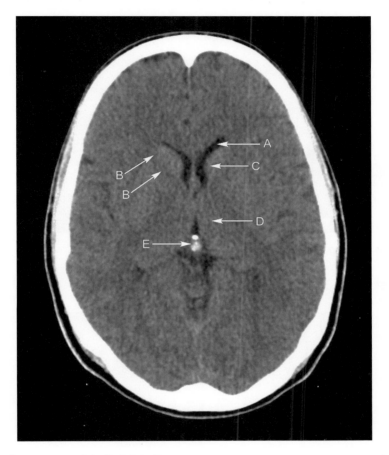

Name the structures labelled **A** to **E**.

Question 1.2

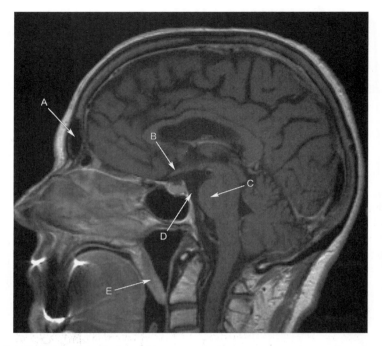

Name the structures labelled A to E.

Question 1.3   This is an axial ultrasound of the neck.

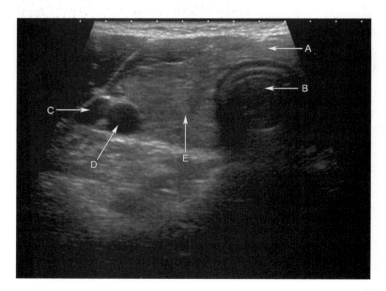

Name the structures labelled **A** to **E**.

Question 1.4

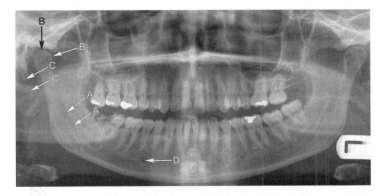

Name the structures labelled **A** to **D**.
E What passes through the structure labelled D?

Question 1.5

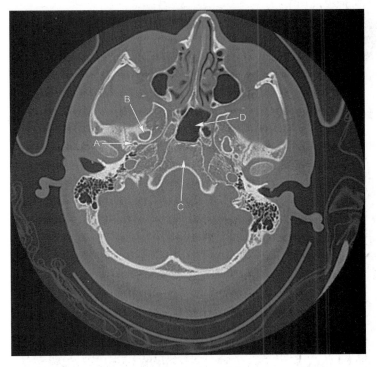

Name the structures labelled **A** to **D**.
E What artery passes through A?

Question 1.6

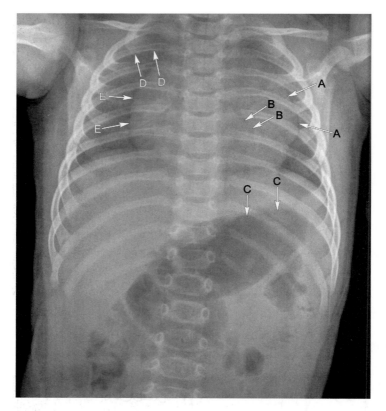

Name the structures labelled **A** to **E**.

Question 1.7

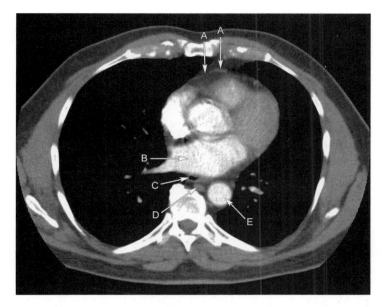

Name the structures labelled **A** to **E**.

Question 1.8

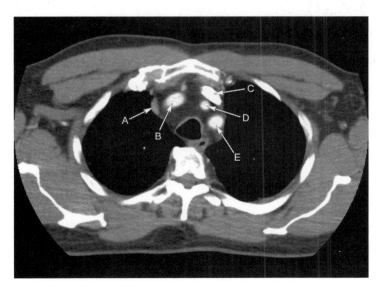

Name the structures labelled **A** to **E**.

Question 1.9

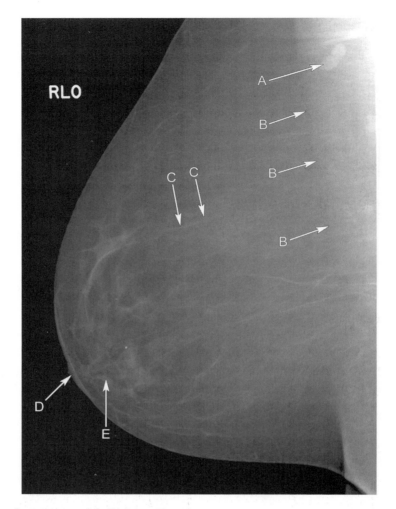

RLO

Name the structures labelled **A** to **E**.

Question 1.10   This is a transverse pelvic ultrasound in a 30-year-old woman.

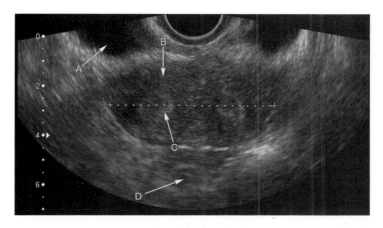

Name the structures labelled **A** to **D**.
E What normal variant is present?

Question 1.11

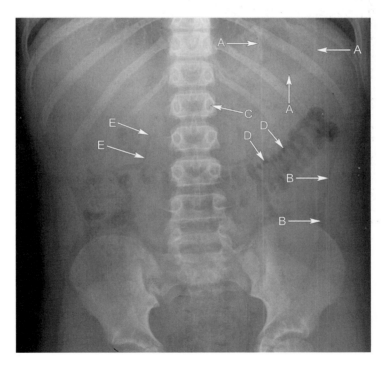

Name the structures labelled **A** to **E**.

Question 1.12 This is a transverse ultrasound of the abdomen.

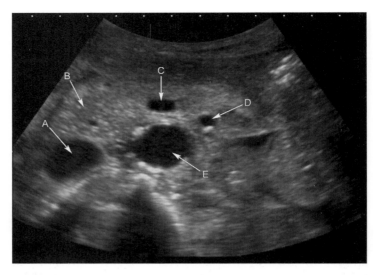

Name the structures labelled **A** to **E**.

Question 1.13

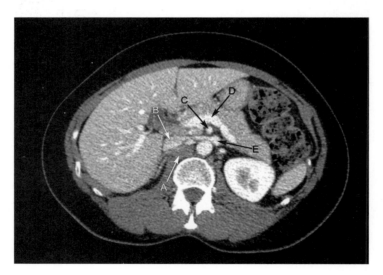

Name the structures labelled **A** to **E**.

Question 1.14

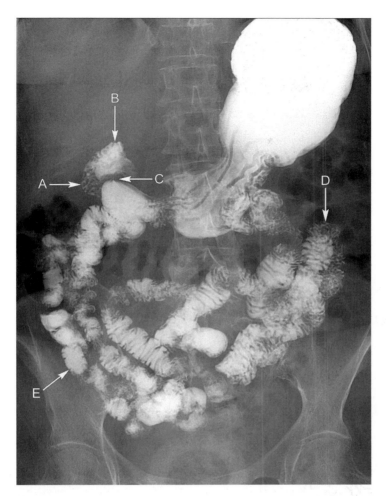

Name the structures labelled **A** to **E**.

Question 1.15

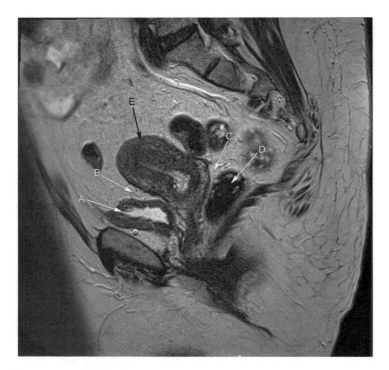

Name the structures labelled **A** to **E**.

Question 1.16

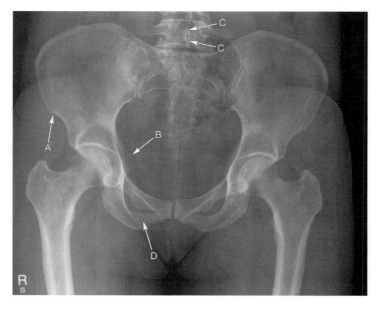

Name the structures labelled **A** to **D**.
E What muscle originates from **A**?

Question 1.17 This is an MRI of the right knee.

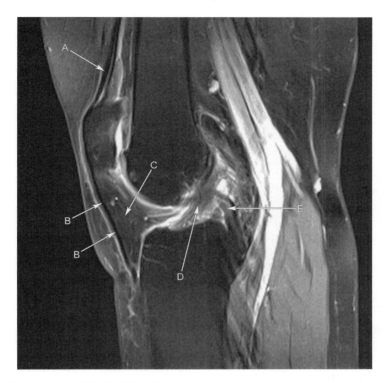

Name the structures labelled **A** to **E**.

Question 1.18   This is an oblique sagittal MRI of the shoulder.

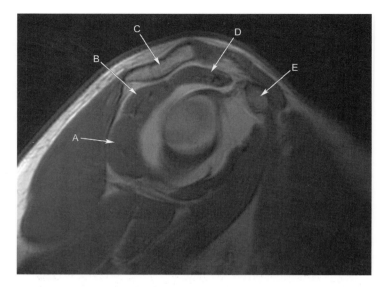

Name the structures labelled **A** to **E**.

Question 1.19

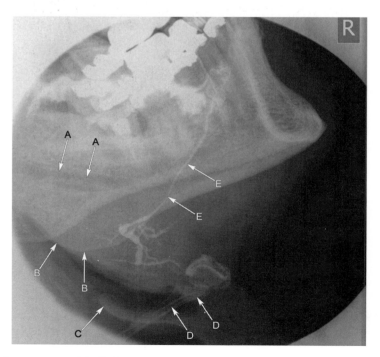

Name the structures labelled **A** to **E**.

Question 1.20

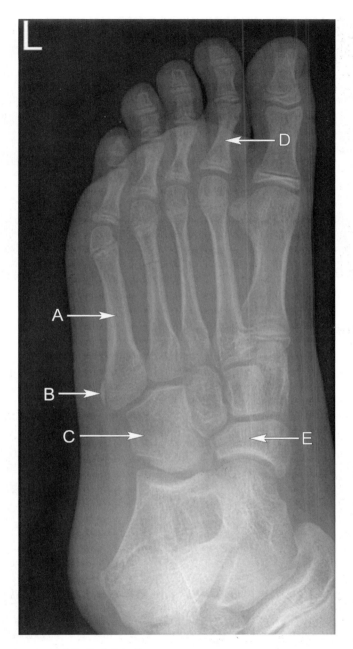

Name the structures labelled **A** to **E**.

Examination 1: Answers

1.1 Axial CT scan of the brain

A Frontal horn of the left lateral ventricle.
B Anterior limb of the right internal capsule.
C Head of the left caudate nucleus.
D Left thalamic nucleus.
E Pineal gland.

The heads of the caudate nuclei are located in the concavities of the frontal horns of the lateral ventricles. The internal capsule lies lateral to the caudate nucleus and is split into anterior and posterior limbs. The anterior limb is located between the caudate nucleus and the globus pallidus of the lentiform nucleus. There are two thalami, which are located lateral to the third ventricle and medially to the posterior limb of the internal capsule. The pineal gland is a midline structure located posterior to the third ventricle and is often calcified.

1.2 Sagittal T1 MRI scan of the brain

A Frontal sinus.
B Optic chiasm.
C Pons.
D Prepontine cistern.
E Soft palate.

The paired frontal sinuses lie superior to the nose and orbits and are located between the inner and outer tables of the frontal bone. The two optic nerves partially decussate at the optic chiasm in the middle cranial fossa. The brainstem consists of the medulla oblongata, pons and midbrain. The pons can be recognized on sagittal imaging by its bulging anterior surface, in front of which is the prepontine cistern (one of the subarachnoid basal cisterns, located between the pons and the clivus). The palate forms the roof of the mouth and is formed by the soft and hard palates. The posterior third (fibromuscular part) forms the soft palate and the anterior two-thirds (bony part) forms the hard palate.

1.3 Transverse ultrasound of the thyroid gland

A Isthmus of thyroid gland.
B Trachea.
C Right internal jugular vein.
D Right common carotid artery.
E Right lobe of the thyroid gland.

The thyroid gland consists of two lobes joined by a central isthmus. Each lobe is divided into an upper and lower pole. The central isthmus lies anterior to the trachea at the level of C6. The carotid sheath lies posterolaterally to the thyroid lobes and contains the internal jugular vein (laterally), common carotid artery (medially) and the vagus nerve (not visualized on ultrasound).

1.4 Orthopantomogram (OPG)

A Right inferior alveolar canal.
B Right mandibular condyle.
C Right styloid process.
D Right mental foramen.
E Right mental nerve.

The mandible is made up of two halves, each half consisting of a body, an angle, a ramus, a coronoid process and a condylar neck and process. The condylar process forms the mandibular portion of the temporomandibular joint and articulates with the temporal bone. The mental foramen is the exit foramen for the inferior alveolar nerve (a branch of the mandibular division of the trigeminal nerve (CN V^3)). The styloid process of the temporal bone lies anterior to the mastoid process and is the origin for the stylohyoid muscle.

1.5 Axial CT of the base of the skull

A Right foramen spinosum.
B Right foramen ovale.
C Clivus.
D Sphenoid sinus.
E Right middle meningeal artery.

The foramen spinosum transmits the middle meningeal artery. The foramen ovale transmits the mandibular division (CN V^3) of the trigeminal nerve and the accessory meningeal artery. The sphenoid sinuses are a pair of sinuses whose relations are as follows:

Anteriorly	Ethmoid air cells
Posteriorly	Clivus
Superiorly	Sella turcica
Inferiorly	Nasopharynx
Laterally	Cavernous sinus

The base of the skull and the contents of the foramina are a common exam topic and the following table should be learnt:

Foramina	Contents
Foramen ovale	Mandibular division of the trigeminal nerve (CN V^3) Accessory meningeal artery
Carotid canal	Internal carotid artery Sympathetic plexus
Jugular foramen	Internal jugular vein Glossopharyngeal nerve (CN IX) Vagus nerve (CN X) Accessory nerve (CN XI)
Stylomastoid foramen	Facial nerve (CN VII) Stylomastoid artery
Foramen spinosum	Middle meningeal artery and vein
Foramen lacerum	Internal carotid artery
Foramen magnum	Medulla and surrounding meninges Spinal roots of the accessory nerve Anterior and posterior spinal and vertebral arteries

1.6 AP X-ray of the neonatal chest

A Thymus.
B Left lower lobe bronchus.
C Stomach.
D Posterior right third rib.
E Thymus.

The neonatal chest X-ray (CXR) is performed as a supine antero-posterior radiograph that exaggerates the heart size and mediastinal width. The normal evolution of the CXR appearances from neonates to adults should be understood in order to recognize pathology when present. For instance, it is normal to see the thymus gland on neonatal CXR but in adults this should not be visualized.

The thymus is a specialized organ for the production of T-lymphocytes of the immune system. It is located in the anterior superior mediastinum and is most prominent in the neonatal period. As the child grows, it becomes much less prominent on CXR and after about eight years old it is not readily identifiable.

Aids to recognition of the thymus gland include:

- Its characteristic 'sail' shape.
- Location in the anterior mediastinum should not obscure the heart borders.
- Scalloping of the border of the thymus by the anterior ribs.
- A normal thymus will not displace the trachea: if this is identified, another pathology must be suspected.

1.7 Axial CT chest with contrast

A Pericardium.
B Left atrium.
C Oesophagus.
D Azygos vein.
E Descending thoracic aorta.

The pericardium consists of visceral and parietal layers, envelops the heart and great vessels and is seen on axial CT as a thin dense line separated from the myocardium by epicardial fat. The azygos vein commences at the level of L2 and ascends anteriorly to the vertebral bodies of the thoracic vertebrae up to the level of T4 and to the right of the descending thoracic aorta. At T4, the azygos vein crosses superior to the right hilum and drains into the superior vena cava. The left atrium lies anterior to the oesophagus, which explains why left atrial enlargement can cause dysphagia.

1.8 Axial CT chest with contrast

A Right brachiocephalic (innominate) vein.
B Brachiocephalic (innominate) artery.
C Left brachiocephalic (innominate) vein.
D Left common carotid artery.
E Left subclavian artery.

From right to left, the branches of the arch of the aorta are the brachiocephalic artery, left common carotid artery and left subclavian artery. The left common carotid and left subclavian arteries lie to the left of the trachea. All three branches are crossed anteriorly by the left brachiocephalic vein. The brachiocephalic veins are formed by the union of the subclavian and internal jugular veins. The right brachiocephalic vein lies to the far right side of the great vessels.

1.9 Medial lateral oblique mammogram of the right breast

A Right axillary lymph node.
B Right pectoralis major muscle.
C Ligament of Astley Cooper (suspensory ligament of the right breast).
D Right nipple.
E Right retroareolar duct.

Retroareloar ducts radiate from the nipple and are visible in the older age group of women, owing to the replacement of glandular tissue with fatty tissue. The ligaments of Astley Cooper are connective tissue of the breast that run from the deep fascia and maintain the structure of the breast. Distortion and thickening of the ligaments can help to identify breast malignancies.

1.10 Transverse transvaginal ultrasound of the female pelvis

A Bladder.
B Myometrium.
C Endometrium.
D Rectum.
E Bicornuate uterus.

The uterus is well demonstrated on transvaginal ultrasound, which is the primary modality for imaging the female reproductive organs. It is located between the bladder and the rectum. The inner thin echogenic layer of the uterus is called the endometrium and the outer less echogenic muscular layer is called the myometrium. This image demonstrates a bicornuate uterus (literally translated as a uterus with two horns) where the inferior aspect of the uterus is normal and the superior aspect is bifurcated giving the uterus a heart shaped appearance.
  Other uterine abnormalities include:

Uterine didelphus	The patient has a double uterus
Uterine septum	A septum that splits the uterus into two parts
Unicornuate uterus	Only one side of the uterus forms, giving the uterus a 'penis' shape

1.11 AP X-ray of the abdomen

A Stomach.
B Left properitoneal fat stripe/line.
C Left pedicle of L1.
D Transverse colon.
E Right psoas shadow/outline.

The properitoneal fat stripe represents the layer of fat that separates the peritoneum from the muscles of the anterior abdominal wall. Loss of the stripe may indicate pathology within the abdomen, such as peritonitis. The large bowel can be differentiated from the small bowel by its peripheral location and mucosal markings with haustra only crossing two-thirds of the bowel wall. The psoas major originates from the transverse processes, vertebral bodies and intervertebral discs of T12–L5 and is defined on the abdominal radiograph by a thin radiolucent fat line. The line may be missing in normal individuals. However, asymmetry of the lines may indicate retro-peritoneal pathology, such as haemorrhage, abscess or tumour.

1.12 Transverse ultrasound of the abdomen

A Inferior vena cava.
B Head of the pancreas.
C Superior mesenteric vein.
D Superior mesenteric artery.
E Aorta.

The inferior vena cava (IVC) lies to the right of the abdominal aorta. The superior mesenteric vein lies to the right of the superior mesenteric artery. The superior mesenteric artery can also be differentiated from the vein on ultrasound as its wall is more echogenic. The superior mesenteric vein and artery run between the neck and body of the pancreas anteriorly and the uncinate process of the pancreas posteriorly. The left renal vein can sometimes be seen at this level, crossing the aorta anteriorly to drain into the inferior vena cava.

1.13 Axial CT abdomen with IV contrast

A Right crus of the diaphragm.
B Inferior vena cava.
C Superior mesenteric artery.
D Splenic vein.
E Left renal vein.

The crura of the diaphragm are tendinous structures that attach the diaphragm to the vertebral column. The right crus is larger and longer than the left and is attached to L1, L2 and L3. Because the inferior vena cava is on the right of the aorta, the left renal vein is longer than the right and passes anterior to the aorta. The left renal vein receives:

• Gonadal vein (testicular in males, ovarian in females).
• Left inferior phrenic vein.
• Left suprarenal vein.
• Left second lumbar vein.

These vessels drain directly into the inferior vena cava on the right side.
    The superior mesenteric artery arises from the anterior surface of the aorta, just inferior to the origin of the coeliac trunk, at the vertebral level of L1. It supplies the intestine from the distal duodenum to the distal two-thirds of the transverse colon. The splenic vein runs posterior to the body and neck of the pancreas to join the superior mesenteric vein that together form the portal vein.

1.14 Barium follow-through

A Second part of the duodenum.
B Duodenal cap.
C Pylorus of the stomach.
D Jejunum.
E Distal ileum.

The duodenum is composed of four parts: it connects the stomach to the jejunum, beginning at the duodenal cap and ending at the duodenal jejunal (DJ) flexure, where it is supported by the ligament of Treitz. The DJ flexure normally lies to the left of the midline in the transpyloric plane, and its location is important in the diagnosis of malrotation of the small bowel. The first three parts of the duodenum form a 'C' shape, within which the head of the pancreas lies within the concavity of the 'C'. The pancreatic and common bile ducts enter into the ampulla of Vater in the second part of the duodenum. Only the proximal aspect of the first part of the duodenum is intraperitoneal with the remainder of the duodenum in the retro-peritoneal space.

The proximal two-fifths of the small intestine are called the jejunum and the distal three-fifths, the ileum. They can be distinguished on a barium follow-through by:

- Location (the jejunum is found in the left upper abdomen).
- Mucosal folds (thicker and more prominent valvulae conniventes in the jejunum).
- Lymphoid follicles or Peyer's patches (more numerous in the ileum).

1.15 Sagittal T2 MRI of the female pelvis

A Bladder.
B Vesicouterine pouch.
C Pouch of Douglas (rectouterine pouch).
D Rectum.
E Uterine fundus.

The uterus is pear-shaped and composed of four parts: the fundus, body, cervix and internal os. It lies between the rectum and the bladder. The rectouterine pouch (pouch of Douglas) is an extension of the peritoneal cavity between the posterior uterus and the anterior rectum and is a common site for the spread of pathology and collection of fluid. The rectum is the final portion of the large intestine and is about 12 cm long. The lower third of the rectum is extraperitoneal. The levator ani supports the vis-cera and together with the coccygeus forms the pelvic floor. It is composed of three muscles: the puborectalis, pubococcygeus and iliococcygeus.

1.16 AP X-ray of the pelvis

A Right anterior inferior iliac spine.
B Right ischial spine.
C Spinous process of L5.
D Right inferior pubic ramus.
E Right rectus femoris muscle.

The pelvis is formed by the sacrum and coccyx posteriorly and the two hip bones laterally and anteriorly. The hip bones are composed of the pubis, ischium and ilium. The anterior inferior iliac spine is the origin for the rectus femoris and is a recognized site for avulsion fractures. The ischium is situated inferiorly to the ilium and posteriorly to the pubis. The ischial tuberosity is the origin for the hamstring muscles and is another recognized site for avulsion fractures. The ischial spine is a triangular bony eminence to which the levator ani and sacrospinous ligament are attached.

1.17 Sagittal proton density MRI of the right knee

A Quadriceps tendon.
B Patella tendon.
C Hoffa's fat pad (infrapatellar fat pad).
D Anterior cruciate ligament.
E Posterior cruciate ligament.

The quadriceps tendon connects the quadriceps muscles to the superior surface of the patella. The patella tendon connects the inferior surface of the patella to the tibial tuberosity. Like the fibres of external oblique muscle in the anterior abdominal wall, the direction of the fibres of the anterior cruciate ligament can be remembered by the analogy of 'hands in your pockets', originating from the medial surface of the lateral femoral condyle to attach anterior to the intercondyloid eminence of the tibia. The fibres of the posterior cruciate ligament run in the opposite direction to the anterior cruciate ligament and extend from the posterior intercondylar area of the tibia to the lateral surface of the medial femoral condyle.

The infrapatellar fat pad (Hoffa's fat pad) is an intracapsular structure situated posterior to the patellar tendon and is routinely visualized on MRI of the knee. It is important to be familiar with its appearance, as it can be commonly injured and may be the only site of pathology.

1.18 Sagittal MRI T1 arthrogram of the right shoulder

A Right teres minor muscle.
B Right infraspinatus muscle.
C Right acromion.
D Right supraspinatus muscle.
E Right coracoid process.

Stability of the hip is provided mainly by the bony acetabulum. Stability of the shoulder is provided by a group of four muscles that together form the rotator cuff. The muscles of the rotator cuff can be remembered using the mnemonic **SITS**:

- **S**upraspinatous.
- **I**nfraspinatous.
- **T**eres minor.
- **S**ubscapularis.

The teres minor and infraspinatus are external rotators of the shoulder. The teres minor originates from the dorsal surface of the axillary border of the scapula and inserts onto the greater tuberosity of the shoulder. The infraspinatus originates from the infraspinous fossa of the scapula and is also attached to the greater tuberosity of the shoulder. The acromion is the distal continuation of the spine of the scapula, extends laterally over the shoulder joint and articulates with the clavicle to form the acromioclavicular joint. The supraspinatus initiates abduction of the shoulder and originates from the supraspinatus fossa of the scapula, passing immediately inferior to the acromion and inserting into the greater tuberosity of the humerus. The coracoid is a bony anterior eminence of the scapula and provides a useful landmark for identifying the anterior structures when assessing sagittal cross-sectional imaging of the shoulder. If the coracoid is on your **RIGHT** as you look at the image on a sagittal section of the shoulder then you are looking at the **RIGHT** shoulder.

1.19 Submandibular sialogram

A Right inferior alveolar canal.
B Angle of the right mandible.
C Epiglottis.
D Hyoid bone.
E Right Wharton's duct (submandibular duct).

Sialograms of the salivary glands are performed to assess the salivary ducts for flow, obstruction and filling defects (e.g., calculi). A cannula is inserted into the relevant duct opening within the mouth, contrast is injected and radiographs taken. Standard views are an AP view and a lateral oblique view of the examined side. A right lateral oblique X-ray is therefore performed for imaging the right submandibular gland.

The submandibular ducts (Wharton's ducts) open into the anterior floor of the mouth, under the tongue and on either side of the frenulum linguae. The parotid ducts (Stenson's ducts) open into the rear of the mouth opposite the upper second molar tooth. The inferior alveolar canal transmits the inferior alveolar nerve (a terminal branch of the mandibular division of the trigeminal nerve (CN V³)) and exits the mandible via the mental foramen, where it supplies the sensation to the chin and lower lip. It is at risk of injury during the removal of wisdom teeth.

1.20 Oblique X-ray of the left foot

A Diaphysis of the left fifth metatarsal.
B Left os vesalianum.
C Left cuboid.
D Diaphysis of the proximal phalanx of the left second toe.
E Left navicular.

The cuboid is one of the seven tarsal bones of the foot. It articulates proximally with the calcaneum to from the calcaneocuboid joint and distally with the fourth and fifth metatarsals. The navicular is located on the medial side of the foot and articulates proximally with the talus, laterally with the cuboid and distally with the three cuneiform bones.

Accessory bones are normal variants and will arise in the exam. The os vesalianum is an accessory bone located proximal to the base of the fifth metatarsal, and is found within the peroneus brevis tendon. It should be remembered as a normal variant, as it is commonly confused with a fracture of the base of the fifth metatarsal.

Other common accessory variants found in the foot are:

Os peroneum	Located laterally to the cuboid
	Associated with the peroneus longus tendon
Os tibiale externum or os naviculare	An accessory navicular
	Located adjacent to the medial side of the navicular and within the tendon of tibialis posterior
Os supranaviculare	Located superior to the navicular
Os trigonum	Located posterior to the talus

For further information on the accessory ossicles of the foot, see Question 10.19.

Examination 2: Questions

Question 2.1

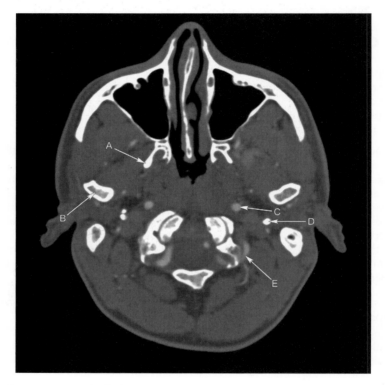

Name the structures labelled **A** to **E**.

Question 2.2

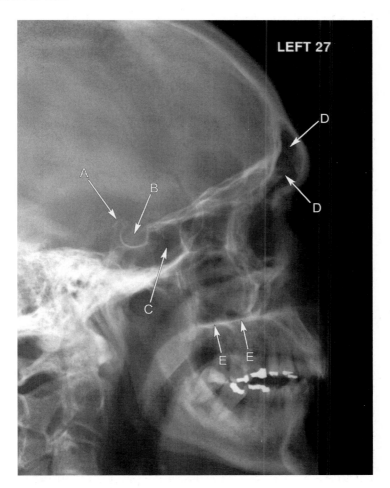

Name the structures labelled **A** to **E**.

Question 2.3

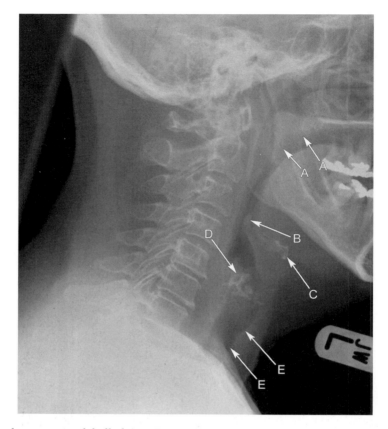

Name the structures labelled **A** to **E**.

Question 2.4

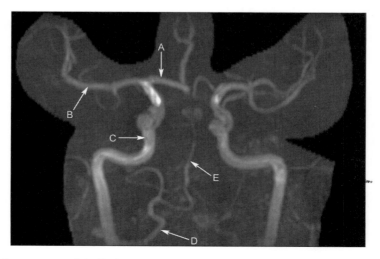

Name the structures labelled **A** to **E**.

Question 2.5

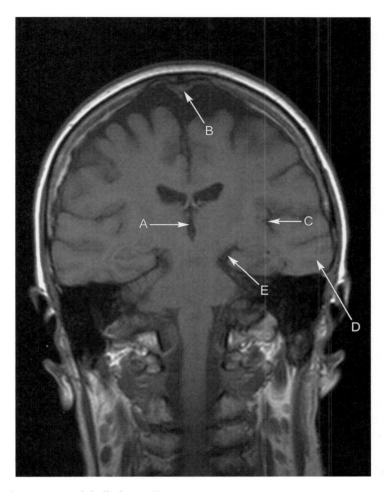

Name the structures labelled **A** to **E**.

Question 2.6

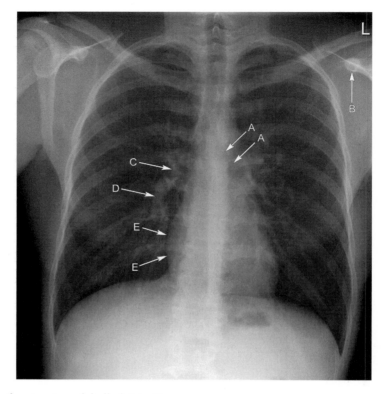

Name the structures labelled **A** to **D**.
E Which cardiac chamber makes up this part of the cardiac silhouette?

Question 2.15

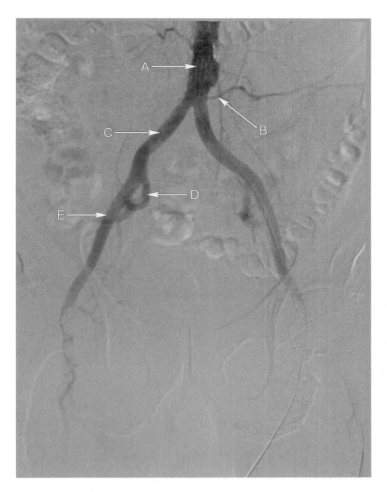

Name the structures labelled **A** to **E**.

Question 2.16

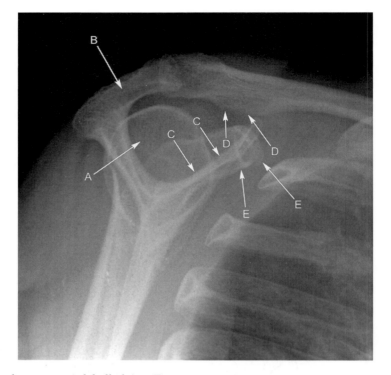

Name the structures labelled **A** to **E**.

Question 2.17

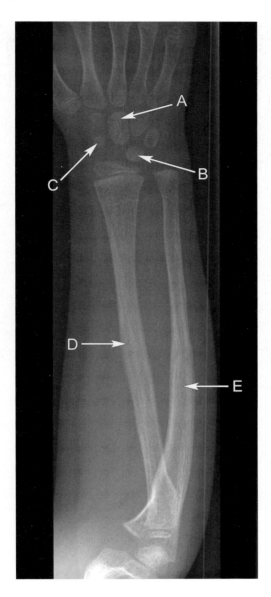

This is a radiograph of right forearm.
Name the structures labelled **A** to **E**.

Question 2.18

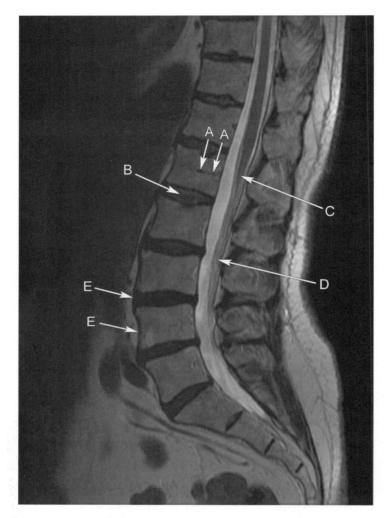

Name the structures labelled **A** to **E**.

Question 2.19

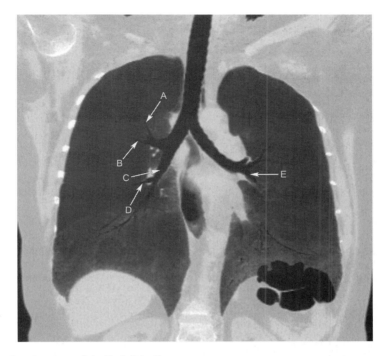

Name the structures labelled **A** to **E**.

Question 2.20

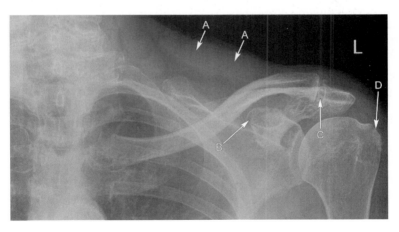

Name the structures labelled **A** to **D**.
E Which three ligaments attach to B?

Examination 2: Answers

2.1 Axial CT of the upper neck with IV contrast

A Right lateral pterygoid plate.
B Right mandibular condyle.
C Left internal carotid artery.
D Left styloid process.
E Left vertebral artery.

The lateral and medial pterygoid plates are part of the sphenoid bone and descend perpendicularly from the region where the body and the greater wings unite. All categories of Le Fort fracture involve the pterygoid plates. The internal carotid artery arises at the level of C3 (where the common carotid artery bifurcates) and enters the base of the skull through the carotid canal. The styloid process is a pointed thin piece of bone that extends from the inferior surface of the temporal bone and serves as an important attachment to several ligaments and muscles of the larynx and tongue. The vertebral arteries are paired arteries that usually arise from the subclavian arteries and course through the foramen transversarium from C6 to C1. This image demonstrates the path of the vertebral arteries as they enter the foramen magnum, where they unite to form the basilar artery.

2.2 Lateral X-ray of the skull

A Posterior clinoid process.
B Sella turcica (pituitary fossa).
C Sphenoid sinus.
D Frontal sinus.
E Hard palate.

The sella turcica is a depression within the sphenoid bone that houses the pituitary gland. The anterior border is formed by two small bony eminences called the anterior clinoid processes. The posterior border is formed by a flat square piece of bone called the dorsum sellae, from which two small bony eminences arise called the posterior clinoid processes. These not only deepen the sella but also form the attachment for the tentorium cerebelli. The sphenoid sinuses are paired sinuses within the body of the sphenoid bone. The hard palate forms the anterior two-thirds of the roof of the mouth, separating the mouth from the nasal cavity.

2.3 Lateral X-ray of the cervical spine

A Soft palate.
B Epiglottis.
C Hyoid bone.
D Thyroid cartilage.
E Trachea.

The soft palate forms the posterior third of the roof of the mouth. The epiglottis is a flap of elastic cartilage, which protects the glottis during swallowing. When enlarged in patients with epiglottitis, the epiglottis gives the characteristic 'thumb-print' sign. The hyoid bone is a horseshoe-shaped bone located between the mandible and the thyroid cartilage at the level of C3. It is the only bone in the body that does not articulate with another bone. The cricoid cartilage is situated inferior to the thyroid cartilage at the level of C6 and is the only complete ring of cartilage around the trachea. The trachea extends from the larynx (at the level of C5) to the carina (T4/5) and, apart from the cricoid cartilage, is surrounded by incomplete C-shaped rings of cartilage.

A recap of levels on the lateral C-spine:

Level	Structure
C3	Hyoid bone
	Bifurcation of the common carotid arteries
C5	Trachea
C6	Cricoid cartilage
	Commencement of the oesophagus

2.4 MR angiogram of the circle of Willis

A Right anterior cerebral artery.
B Right middle cerebral artery.
C Right internal carotid artery.
D Right vertebral artery.
E Basilar artery.

The circle of Willis is a pentagonal arterial circle and comprises of, from posterior to anterior:

- Posterior cerebral arteries, making the back wall.
- Posterior communicating arteries, making the posterior side walls.
- Internal carotid arteries, making the corners.
- Anterior cerebral arteries, making the anterior side walls.
- Anterior communicating artery, making the tip and connecting the anterior cerebral arteries.

The basilar artery, which is formed by the two vertebral arteries, divides into the posterior cerebral arteries and is not considered part of the circle.

For a diagram of the circle of Willis see Question 5.2.

2.5 Coronal T1 MRI of the brain

A Third ventricle.
B Superior sagittal sinus.
C Left sylvian fissure.
D Left temporal lobe.
E Left ambient cistern.

The surface of the cerebral hemispheres is divided with fissures and sulci. Fissures involve the entire thickness of the cerebral wall, while sulci only affect the surface of the wall. The sylvian fissure lies superior to the temporal lobe and divides the frontal and parietal lobe. It is an important landmark when reviewing area on CT scans to look for evidence of subarachnoid haemorrhage.

Cisterns are cerebrospinal-fluid-filled subarachnoid spaces in the brain. Starting from inferiorly to superiorly these are:

Cisterna magna	Also known as the cerebellomedullary cistern The largest of the cisterns and located between the posterior surface of the medulla oblongata and the cerebellum
Prepontine cistern	Located anterior to the pons
Suprasellar cistern	The cistern located just superior to the pituitary fossa Continuous posteriorly with the interpeduncular cistern
Interpeduncular cistern	Located between the cerebral peduncles Continuous anteriorly with the suprasellar cistern and inferiorly with the prepontine cistern
Ambient cistern	Basically, a thin extension of the quadrigeminal cistern Extends laterally from the quadrageminal cistern around the midbrain of the brainstem to connect to the interpeduncular cistern
Quadrigeminal cistern	Also known as the superior cistern or the cistern of the great cerebral vein as it contains the great cerebral vein Located between the superior surface of the cerebellum and the splenium of the corpus callosum
Cistern of the velum interpositum	Also known as the cavum velum interpositum A triangular space seen on axial CT Located just superior to the quadragminal cistern, with which it is continuous

2.6 PA X-ray of the chest

A Left main bronchus.
B Left coracoid process.
C Right hilum or hilar point.
D Right interlobar pulmonary artery.
E Right atrium.

The pulmonary arteries, veins and bronchi make up the hila. The hilar point is formed by the descending upper lobe veins superiorly as they cross behind the interlobar pulmonary artery inferiorly. The angle between the vessels is known as the hilar angle and normally measures 120°. The right hilar point is normally located 1 cm lower than the left hilar point and should never be located higher than the left. The left heart border consists of the left atrium superiorly and left ventricle inferiorly. The right heart border consists of the right atrium alone.

2.7 Coronal CT of the chest with IV contrast

A Right vertebral artery.
B Right thyrocervical trunk.
C Right subclavian artery.
D Aortic arch.
E Pulmonary trunk.

The arch of the aorta commences at T4/5, which is also the level of the third costal cartilage. It reaches the T3/4 level at its apex and ends at the T4 level. It runs posteriorly from right to left, passing anterior to the trachea and over the left main bronchus and left main pulmonary artery. There are three main branches of the aortic arch. From right to left these are the brachiocephalic, left common carotid and left subclavian arteries. The right subclavian artery arises from the brachiocephalic artery.

The subclavian artery is divided into three parts as defined by the scalenus anterior. The first part is from the vessel's origin to the medial border of the scalenus anterior. The second part lies posterior to the scalenus anterior and the third part is from the lateral border of the scalenus anterior to the inferior border of the first rib (where the artery becomes the axillary artery). The first branch of the first part of the subclavian artery is the vertebral artery, which ascends to the brain through the foramen transversarium of the cervical vertebrae. The second branch of the first part of the subclavian artery is the thyrocervical trunk.

2.8 Axial CT of the neck with IV contrast

A Right vallecula.
B Median glossoepiglottic fold.
C Hyoid bone.
D Epiglottis.
E Left sternocleidomastoid muscle.

The epiglottic valleculae are depressions found just posterior to the base of the tongue and anterior to the epiglottis. Mucous membranes cover the anterior surface of the epiglottis. These are reflected from the epiglottis to the lateral walls of the pharynx and the root of the tongue, where they are called the glossoepiglottic folds. These comprise one median fold (as demonstrated) and two lateral folds.

The sternocleidomastoid muscle is a paired muscle located in the anterior superficial layers of the neck and is named after its bony attachments – the manubrium (sterno), clavicle (cleido) and mastoid processes of the temporal bone. The sternocleidomastoid can be recognized on CT as it is superficially related to the carotid sheath (as demonstrated in this image with the vessels filled with contrast). The carotid artery can be identified as it lies medial to the internal jugular vein.

The characteristic horseshoe shape of the hyoid bone is well demonstrated on axial CT and lies at the level of C3 between the mandible and the thyroid cartilage. It is the only bone in the body that does not articulate with any other bone and provides an important attachment for the muscles of pharynx posteriorly, the muscles of the floor of the mouth and tongue superiorly and the larynx inferiorly.

2.9 Axial CT of the chest with IV contrast

A Sternum.
B Right superior pulmonary vein.
C Right latissimus dorsi.
D Oesophagus.
E Superior vena cava.

Latissimus dorsi literally translated in Latin means 'broadest muscle of the back'. It is a large triangular muscle, and is supplied by the thoracodorsal nerve, a branch of the brachial plexus derived from the C6–8 nerves.

There are four pulmonary veins (two from each lung) that carry oxygenated blood from the lungs to the left atrium. These are:

- Right superior pulmonary vein.
- Right inferior pulmonary vein.
- Left superior pulmonary vein.
- Left inferior pulmonary vein.

At the level of the lung roots, the pulmonary veins lie inferior to the pulmonary arteries. The left atrium receives the four pulmonary veins and forms the posterior structure of the heart, lying anterior to the descending thoracic aorta and oesophagus.

2.10 Coronal STIR MRI of the neck

A Right sternocleidomastoid muscle.
B Odontoid peg.
C Pons.
D Left parotid gland.
E Left lateral mass of C1.

The pons is part of the brain stem and lies between the midbrain and the medulla oblongata. It can be recognized on axial and sagittal imaging by the broad anterior bulge on axial imaging and the lateral bulge on the coronal imaging. It is connected to the cerebellum by the cerebellar peduncles.

The parotid gland is the largest of the salivary glands. It is located anterior to the ear where it extends over the ramus of the mandible and then inferiorly over the angle of the mandible. The gland is divided into a larger superficial part and a smaller deep part. The facial nerve (CN VII) runs in a plane through the gland superficial to the main intraparotid vessels, the external carotid artery and the retromandibular vein. On MRI the gland has higher signal intensity on T2 and T1 weighted imaging than the surrounding muscle due to the increased water and fat content.

2.11 AP X-ray of the abdomen

A Stomach.
B Right kidney.
C Ascending colon.
D Right lobe of liver.
E Left psoas muscle.

The outline of the kidneys can be seen on an abdominal radiograph. The right kidney is usually slightly lower than the left, owing to the overlying liver. The upper poles of the kidneys are located at approximately the level of T12 and the lower poles at approximately L3. The renal hilum is usually located at the level of L1/2.

2.12 Longitudinal ultrasound of the right kidney

A Renal pyramid.
B Renal sinus.
C Renal cortex.
D Perirenal fat.
E Morison's pouch (hepatorenal recess).

The echogenic layer surrounding the kidney is the perirenal fat. The renal capsule is not well visualized on ultrasound. The grey outer layer of the kidney is made up of the renal cortex and the pyramids. Sometimes the pyramids cannot be clearly visualized but they can be identified on this image as hypoechoic spaces within the renal cortex. The renal sinus is located within the centre of the kidney and is echogenic on ultrasound because of its fat content. The renal sinus contains the calyces, renal pelvis and sinus fat. The hepatorenal recess (Morison's pouch) is a potential space that lies between the upper pole of the right kidney and the liver and normally should not contain fluid. In the context of trauma, the recess is readily identified on a FAST (focused assessment with sonography for trauma) scan in the emergency department and if fluid is identified an emergency laparotomy may be indicated. See Question 9.13 for further imaging of Morison's pouch.

2.13 Longitudinal ultrasound of the left testis

A Head of the epididymis.
B Testicular vein.
C Testicle.
D Scrotal skin.
E Left renal vein.

Each testis is surrounded by a thin layer of peritoneum called the tunica albuginea, which appears as a hyperechoic band on ultrasound. The tunica albuginea is in turn enveloped by the tunica vaginalis, a dense hypoechoic band of fibrous tissue. Peripheral to this layer is the scrotal skin. The mediastinum testis is not demonstrated on this examination but is seen as a thin echogenic band extending through the testis. On ultrasound the epididymis appears isoechoic or slightly more echogenic than the surrounding testis and has a coarser echotexture. The epididymis is composed of a head, body and tail.

The testicular veins are readily identifiable on testicular ultrasound and should not measure more than 3 mm in diameter. The right testicular vein drains directly into the inferior vena cava whereas the left drains into the left renal vein. The longer and more tortuous course of the left renal vein explains why most varicocoeles are left sided. If a left varicocoele is identified during ultrasonography, the left kidney should also be examined to search for a potential renal tumour obstructing venous drainage.

2.14 Axial T2 MRI of the abdomen

A Left rectus abdominis muscle.
B Portal vein.
C Inferior vena cava.
D Aorta.
E Spleen.

The rectus abdominis are paired abdominal muscles extending vertically down the length of the anterior abdominal wall from the xiphisternum to the pubic symphysis. They are separated by a midline band of connective tissue called the linea alba. The spleen is located in the left upper quadrant of the abdomen beneath the ninth and twelfth ribs. In general it has a maximum normal length of 13 cm in adults.

2.15 Angiogram of the distal aorta

A Abdominal aorta.
B Left lumbar artery.
C Right common iliac artery.
D Right internal iliac artery.
E Right external iliac artery.

The abdominal aorta begins at T12. The branches and levels of the abdominal aorta are:

Name of branch	Vertebral level	Number of branches	Supply
Inferior phrenic	T12	1	Diaphragm
Coeliac	T12	1	Liver, abdominal oesophagus, stomach, duodenum, pancreas
Superior mesenteric	L1	1	Duodenum to transverse colon Pancreas
Middle suprarenal	L1	2	Adrenal glands
Renal	L1	2	Kidneys
Gonadal (testicular artery in males, ovarian arteries in females)	L2	2	Testicles in males Ovaries in females
Lumbar	L1–4	4 branches on each side	Abdominal wall muscles, lumbar vertebra, spinal cord
Inferior mesenteric	L3	1	Splenic flexure to rectum
Median sacral	L4	1	Sacrum and coccyx
Common iliac	L4	2	Pelvis and lower limbs

2.16 Y view X-ray of the right shoulder

A Right humerus head.
B Right acromion.
C Spine of the right scapula.
D Right conoid tubercle.
E Right coracoid process.

The Y view shoulder radiograph refers to the Y-shaped appearance of the scapula on this projection. The body of the scapula represents the stem of the Y. The acromion represents the posterior fork of the Y and the coracoid process represents the anterior fork of the Y. The centre of the Y is the glenoid with the humeral head projected over the centre and the shaft of the humerus projected over the stem of the Y. Anterior or posterior dislocation or subluxation can be assessed on the Y view by assessing the relationship of the humeral head to the glenoid.

2.17 AP X-ray of the paediatric right forearm

A Capitate.
B Lunate.
C Scaphoid.
D Radius.
E Ulna.

In the paediatric wrist, the epiphyseal gaps between the carpal bones and between the radius and ulna are normal and must not be confused with ligamental disruption. The gap between the carpal bones within an adult is normally less than 2 mm. Widening of this gap may indicate ligamentous disruption.

Mnemonics for remembering the carpal bones from the proximal to distal row include 'Some Lovers Try Positions That They Cannot Handle', translating as Scaphoid, Lunate, Triquetral, Pisiform, Trapezium, Trapezoid, Capitate and Hamate.

Confusion between the trapezium and the trapezoid can be cleared by remembering trapeziTHUMB, as the trapeziUM articulates with the thUMB.

2.18 Sagittal T2 MRI of the lumbar spine

A Nutrient vessel of L1.
B Nucleus pulposus of the L1/L2 disc.
C Conus medullaris.
D Cauda equina.
E Anterior longitudinal ligament.

T2 sequences of the lumbar spine can be recognized by the high signal intensity of the cerebrospinal fluid. There are seven cervical, twelve thoracic, five lumbar and five sacral vertebrae. The spinal cord termination is called the conus medullaris and is normally located at the level of L1 or L2. The spinal roots that descend from the lower end of the cord are called the cauda equina, which is Latin for 'the horse's tail'.

The spinal ligaments from anterior to posterior are:

Anterior longitudinal ligament	Extends along the anterior vertebral bodies
Posterior longitudinal ligament	Extends along the posterior vertebral bodies
Ligamentum flavum	Connects the laminae of the adjacent vertebrae
Interspinous ligament	Connect the adjoining spinous processes
Supraspinous ligament	Connects the tips of the spinous processes

The intervertebral discs consist of the central nucleus pulposus and the outer fibrous annulus fibrosus.

2.19 Coronal CT of the chest

A Apical segment of the right upper lobe bronchus.
B Anterior segment of the right upper lobe bronchus.
C Bronchus intermedius.
D Right middle lobe bronchus.
E Inferior segment of the left lingular bronchus.

The right main bronchus is shorter, wider and more vertical than the left main bronchus. For this reason there is a predisposition for foreign bodies preferentially to enter the right main bronchus over the left.

The right main bronchus divides into three main bronchi that then subdivide into a total of ten segmental bronchi. The right upper lobe bronchus arises almost immediately after the tracheal bifurcation. The right main bronchus then continues as the bronchus intermedius, which then subdivides into the right lower and middle lobe bronchi.

The left main bronchus divides into two main bronchi that then subdivide into a total of eight segmental bronchi. The left upper lobe bronchus gives off the lingular lobe bronchus, which then subdivides into the superior and inferior lingular bronchi.

Right lung		Left lung	
Main bronchus	Segmental bronchi	Main bronchus	Segmental bronchi
Right upper lobe bronchus	Apical Posterior Anterior	Left upper lobe bronchus	Apicoposterior Anterior Superior lingular Inferior lingular
Right middle lobe bronchus	Lateral Medial		
Right lower lobe bronchus	Apical Anterior Lateral Posterior Medial basal	Left lower lobe bronchi	Apical Anterior Lateral Posterior

2.20 AP X-ray of the left clavicle

A Left trapezius muscle.
B Left coracoid process.
C Left acromioclavicular joint.
D Greater tuberosity of the left humerus.
E Left coracoclavicular, coracoacromial and coracohumeral ligaments.

The AP projection of the clavicle includes the entirety of the clavicle from the medial articulation with the sternum (the sternoclavicular joint) to the lateral articulation with the acromion (the acromioclavicular joint). Many of the major muscle groups of the shoulder and anterior chest wall have attachments to the clavicle, including the deltoid, trapezius and pectoralis major. The subclavian vessels and brachial plexus pass behind the medial portion of the clavicle. The acromioclavicular joint is stabilized by acromioclavicular ligaments with further vertical stability provided by the coracoacromial and the coracoclavicular ligaments. Tears of these ligaments allow the upper limb to fall inferiorly, separating the clavicle from the acromion with subsequent acromioclavicular dislocation.

Examination 3: Questions

Question 3.1

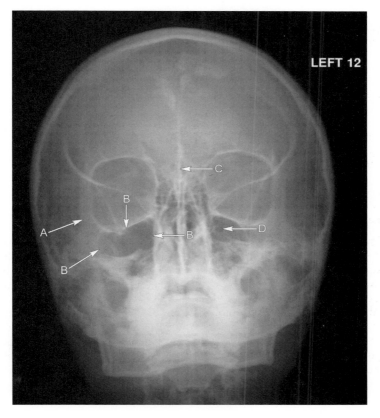

Name the structures labelled **A** to **D**.
E What nerve passes through D?

Question 3.2

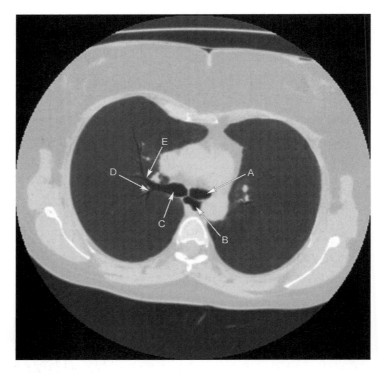

Name the structures labelled **A** to **E**.

Question 3.3

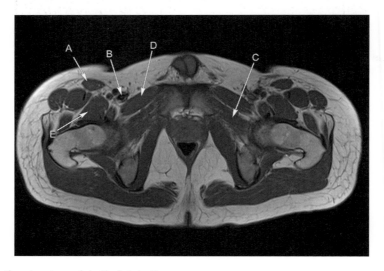

Name the structures labelled **A** to **E**.

Question 3.4

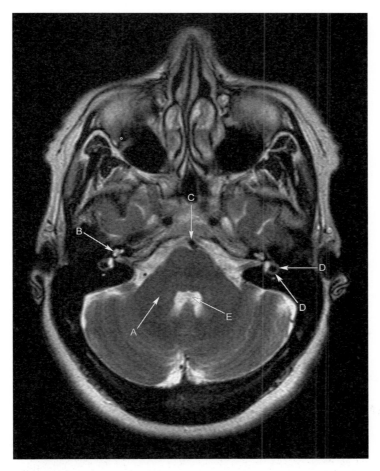

Name the structures labelled **A** to **E**.

Question 3.5

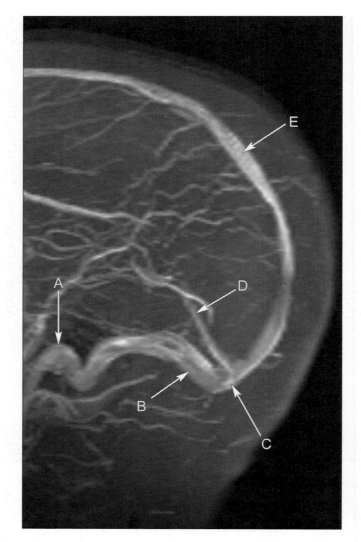

Name the structures labelled **A** to **E**.

Question 3.6

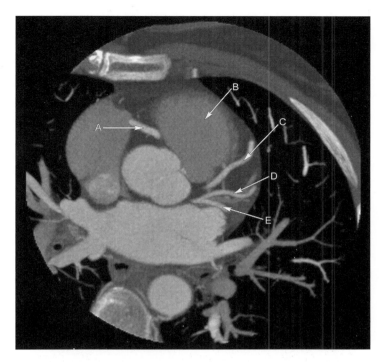

Name the structures labelled **A** to **E**.

Question 3.7

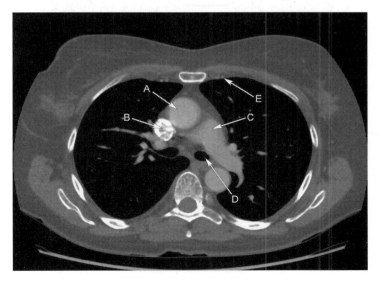

Name the structures labelled **A** to **E**.

Question 3.8

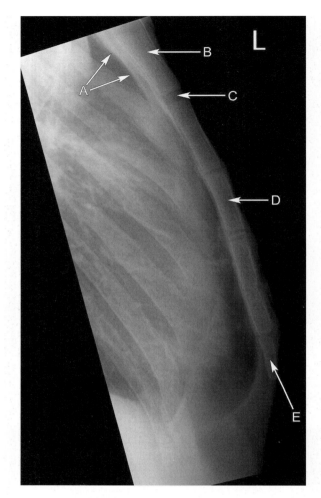

Name the structures labelled **A** to **E**.

Question 3.9

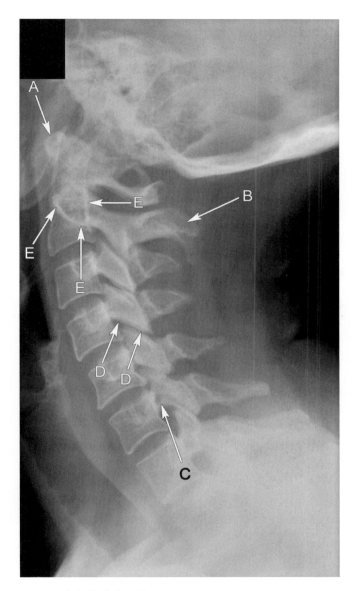

Name the structures labelled **A** to **E**.

Question 3.10

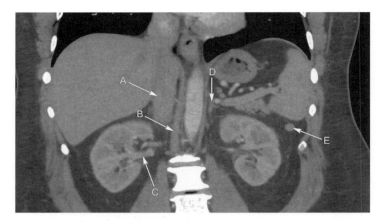

Name the structures labelled **A** to **E**.

Question 3.11

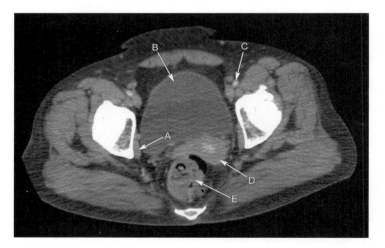

Name the structures labelled **A** to **E**.

Question 3.12

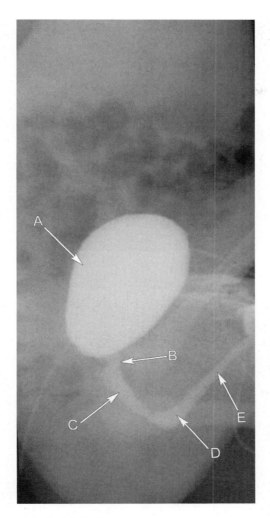

Name the structures labelled **A** to **E**.

Question 3.13

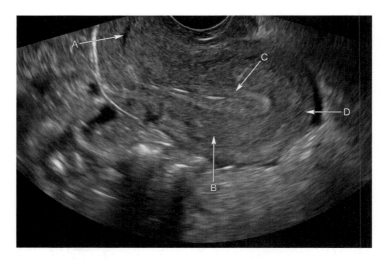

Name the structures labelled **A** to **D**.

E What is the upper limit of normal thickness (mm) of C in a post-menopausal patient?

Question 3.14

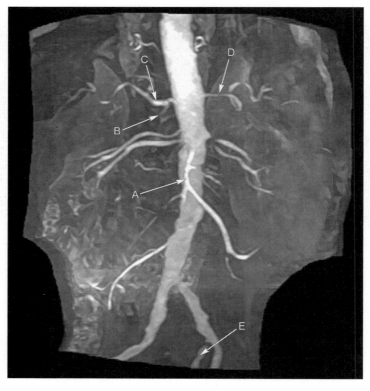

Name the structures labelled **A** to **E**.

Question 3.15

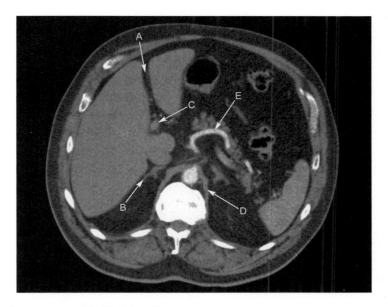

Name the structures labelled **A** to **E**.

Question 3.16

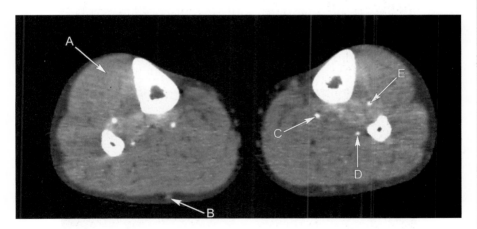

Name the structures labelled **A** to **E**.

Question 3.17

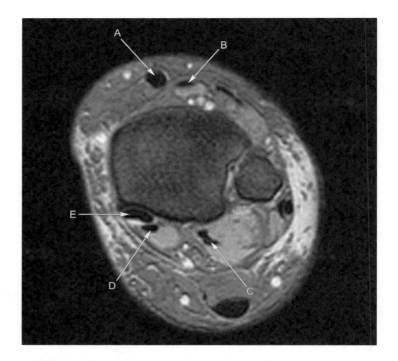

This is an axial MRI of the ankle.
Name the structures labelled **A** to **E**.

Question 3.18

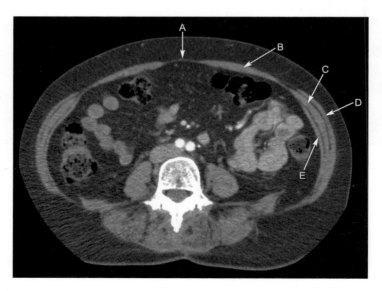

Name the structures labelled **A** to **E**.

Question 3.19

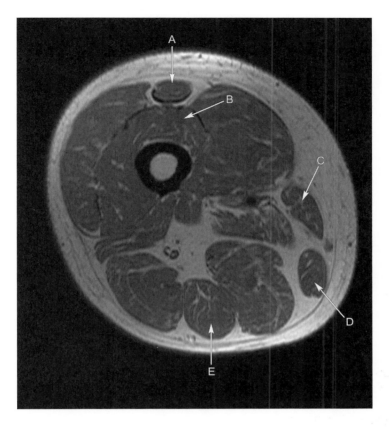

This is an axial MRI of the right thigh.
Name the structures labelled **A** to **E**.

Question 3.20

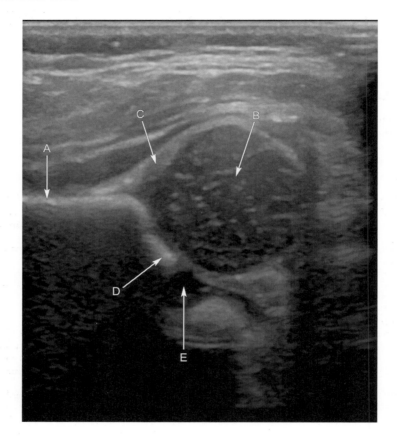

This is an ultrasound of an infant's right hip.
Name the structures labelled **A** to **E**.

Examination 3: Answers

3.1 PA X-ray of the skull

A Frontal process of the right zygomatic bone.
B Right maxillary antrum.
C Crista galli.
D Left foramen rotundum.
E Maxillary branch of the trigeminal nerve.

The trigeminal nerve arises from the lateral surface of the pons and within millimetres enters the trigeminal ganglion, from which three major branches arise and exit the cranium through different foramina. The table below outlines the three divisions:

Division	Exit foramina of the skull	Sensory innervation
Ophthalmic division (V^1)	Superior orbital fissure	Skin of the forehead and superior to the eye
Maxillary division (V^2)	Foramen rotundum, followed by infraorbital foramen	Skin inferior to the eye and superior to the mouth
Mandibular division (V^3)	Foramen ovale	Lower lip, teeth and gums, chin and jaw (also has motor innervation to the muscles of mastication)

The foramen rotundum is projected below the inferior rim of the orbit on facial radiographs and connects the middle cranial fossa with the pterygopalatine fossa. The crista galli is a ridge of bone that extends superiorly from the cribriform plate. It forms the anterior attachment for the falx cerebri. The anterior margin of the lateral orbital wall seen on facial bone radiographs is formed inferiorly by the orbital process of the zygomatic bone and the zygomatic process of the frontal bone superiorly. The junction of these two bones forms the zygomaticofrontal suture.

3.2 Axial CT of the chest

A Left main bronchus.
B Oesophagus.
C Right main bronchus.
D Posterior segment of the right upper lobe bronchus.
E Anterior segment of the right upper lobe bronchus.

The level of this axial section must be demonstrating the upper lobe bronchi as it is above the level of the carina. The right upper lobe bronchus divides into the apical, posterior and anterior subsegmental bronchi. The anterior and posterior subsegmental bronchi are orientated in the transverse plane opposite each other (as demonstrated) whereas the apical branch is orientated vertically. See the answer to Question 2.19 for further detail and a table of the bronchi.

3.3 Axial T1 MRI of the male pelvis

A Right sartorius muscle.
B Right femoral vein.

59

C Left obturator externus muscle.
D Right pectineus muscle.
E Right iliopsoas muscle.

The femoral triangle is an anatomical area of the upper thigh. Its boundaries can be remembered by using the mnemonic **SAIL** – the Sartorius, the Adductor longus and the Inguinal Ligament.

• Medial border – medial border of sartorius.
• Lateral border – medial border of adductor longus.
• Roof – inguinal ligament.

The floor is formed (from lateral to medial) by iliopsoas, pectineus and adductor longus.
    A useful mnemonic for remembering the relative position of the femoral artery, vein and nerve in the groin is **NAVY** (Lateral to medial: Nerve, Artery, Vein, Y-fronts).
    The femoral canal lies medial to the femoral vein, contains the deep inguinal lymph nodes and provides the short narrow passage for femoral herniae.

3.4 Axial T2 MRI of the internal auditory meatus

A Right middle cerebellar peduncle.
B Right cochlea.
C Basilar artery.
D Left lateral semicircular canal.
E Fourth ventricle.

T2 imaging of the brain can be easily recognized by the high signal intensity of the cerebrospinal fluid. MRI has become a primary imaging modality for demonstrating the internal auditory meatus for pathology, such as acoustic neuromas. The seventh and eighth cranial nerves enter the internal acoustic meatus. The cochlea can be recognized as it is fluid filled and therefore has a high signal. For further imaging and description of the internal auditory meatus, see Question 10.3
    The basilar artery lies anterior to the pons in the prepontine cistern and appears black on T2-weighted imaging owing to signal flow void. The cerebellum communicates with the brainstem via the cerebellar peduncles. The fourth ventricle is bounded anteriorly by the pons and upper half of the medulla, posteriorly by the cerebellum and laterally by the cerebellar peduncles. It is continuous with the aqueduct of Sylvius superiorly and the central canal of the spinal cord inferiorly.

3.5 MRI venogram

A Sigmoid sinus.
B Transverse sinus.
C Confluence of the sinuses or torcular herophili.
D Straight sinus.
E Superior sagittal sinus.

The superior sagittal sinus runs from anterior to posterior of the brain, in the midline and between the two cerebral hemispheres, where it enters the confluence of the sinuses (torcular herophili) anterior to the internal occipital protuberance. The straight sinus is formed from the vein of Galen and the inferior sagittal sinus and is well demonstrated on this image, running from the centre of the brain where it drains into the confluence of the sinuses. The right and left transverse sinuses arise from the confluence and drain into respective tortuous sigmoid sinuses before draining into the internal jugular veins at the jugular foramen.
    For a diagram as a further revision aid see Question 4.1

3.6 Axial CTA of the heart

A Right coronary artery.
B Right ventricle.
C Left anterior descending artery.
D Left obtuse marginal artery (M1).
E Left circumflex artery.

There are two main coronary arteries and both arise from the aortic root above the aortic valve. About 4% of people have a third main artery, called the posterior coronary artery.

The right coronary artery originates from the anterior coronary sinus, above the right cusp of the aortic valve. It passes to the right of and posterior to the pulmonary artery. It can be seen emerging from under the right atrial appendage and then coursing along the anterior atrioventricular groove. It first gives rise to a conus branch in 50% of cases and then a sinoatrial branch in 55% of cases (this arises from the left circumflex in the other 45%).

The left coronary artery arises from the left posterior aortic sinus, above the left cusp of the aortic valve. After approximately 5–10 mm, it bifurcates into the left anterior descending artery (which runs down the anterior intraventricular groove to the apex) and the left circumflex artery (which runs in the left posterior atrioventricular groove). The major branches of the left circumflex artery are the obtuse marginal arteries, which are numbered sequentially from proximal to distal. In approximately 15% of cases the left coronary artery trifurcates giving rise to a third branch known as the ramus intermedius artery.

3.7 Axial CT of the chest with IV contrast

A Ascending aorta.
B Superior vena cava.
C Pulmonary trunk.
D Left main bronchus.
E Left internal thoracic artery.

The superior vena cava is formed from the left and right brachiocephalic veins. It is the most lateral of the right-sided mediastinal vessels which makes it particularly susceptible to compression by right upper-lobe tumours and lymphadenopathy. The pulmonary trunk commences from the right atrium, lies to the left of the ascending aorta and divides into the right and left main pulmonary arteries. The right main pulmonary artery is longer than the left as it has to pass under the aortic arch to enter the hilum of the right lung.

3.8 Lateral X-ray of a paediatric sternum

A Parietal pleura.
B Manubrium.
C Manubriosternal joint (angle of Louis).
D Body of sternum.
E Xiphoid process.

The sternum is located in the centre of the thorax and is composed of three parts. The superior part is called the manubrium, the middle is called the body and the inferior part is the xiphoid process. The sternal angle (also called the angle of Louis or the manubriosternal joint) is the angle formed at the junction of the manubrium and the body of the sternum. The angle of Louis lies at the level of the T4/5 and is an important anatomical landmark of the thorax. The mediastinal structures that lie on a horizontal plane with the angle of Louis include:

- The bifurcation of the trachea.
- The start and end of the aortic arch.
- The entry of the azygos vein as it arches over the right main bronchus to enter the trachea.

3.9 Lateral X-ray of the cervical spine

A Anterior arch of C1.
B Spinous process of C2.
C Pedicle of C6.
D Facet joint C4/C5.
E Harris' ring.

C1, C2 and C7 are 'special' vertebrae because each differs from the normal structure of the remaining cervical vertebrae.

- C1 (the atlas) has no vertebral body.
- C2 (the axis) has an odontoid peg.
- C7 (vertebra prominens) has a prominent longer spinous process than the other cervical vertebrae, which is why it is called the vertebra prominens.

3.10 Coronal CT abdomen with IV contrast

A Inferior vena cava.
B Right crus of the diaphragm.
C Right renal vein.
D Left adrenal gland.
E Splenunculus.

The inferior vena cava lies to the right of the aorta and the left renal vein is therefore longer than the right. The left renal vein passes in front of the aorta and the left renal artery. The left renal vein is the drainage pathway for the following veins:

- Left gonadal vein (left testicular vein in males and left ovarian vein in females).
- Left suprarenal vein.
- Left inferior phrenic vein.
- Left second lumbar vein.

The equivalent veins on the right side drain directly into the inferior vena cava.

A splenunculus is a small accessory spleen and commonly appears as a small rounded nodule located near the spleen.

3.11 Axial CT of the female pelvis with IV contrast

A Right obturator internus muscle.
B Bladder.
C Left external iliac artery.
D Uterus.
E Rectum.

The bladder can be recognized on CT not only by its anterior relation to the other pelvic structures but also by its central low (fluid) attenuation.

The obturator internus can be recognized as it 'lines' the pelvic sidewalls. The obturator internus muscle arises from the inner surface of the anterolateral wall of the pelvis. It exits the pelvis through the lesser sciatic foramen to attach to the greater trochanter of the femur.

The rectus abdominis can still be visualized within the anterior abdominal wall and the level of the inguinal ligament has therefore not been reached. It is only when the external iliac artery passes underneath the inguinal ligament that it becomes the common femoral artery. The mnemonic **NAVY** (Nerve, Artery, Vein, Y-fronts) can also be applied to the iliac vessels and nerves, with the external iliac artery lying lateral to the vein.

The rectum is the final part of the colon and is located posterior to the bladder in males and the vagina and uterus in females (the uterus can be seen between the bladder and the rectum in this image).

The sartorius originates from the anterior superior iliac spine and crosses two joints (the hip and the knee) to insert into the medial surface of the tibia. It can be recognized not only as an anterior thigh muscle but because it has a characteristic triangular shape with the tip of the triangle orientated posteriorly.

3.12 Micturating cystourethrogram (MCUG)

A   Bladder.
B   Prostatic urethra.
C   Membranous urethra.
D   Bulbar urethra.
E   Penile urethra.

The MCUG is a dynamic examination for assessing the ureters, bladder and urethra whilst the patient voids. It is commonly indicated for the exclusion of vesicoureteric reflux and posterior urethral valves.

The male urethra is divided into anterior and posterior segments:

Anterior segment	Penile urethra: meatus to the root of the penis Bulbar urethra: root of the penis to the urogenital diaphragm
Posterior segment	Membranous urethra: urogenital diaphragm to the verumontanum of the prostate Prostatic urethra: verumontanum of the prostate to the neck of the bladder

3.13 Longitudinal transvaginal ultrasound of the female pelvis

A   Cervix.
B   Myometrium.
C   Endometrium.
D   Fundus of the uterus.
E   5 mm.

Transvaginal ultrasound provides good imaging of the uterus and is the primary imaging modality for the female reproductive organs. The uterus is a pear-shaped organ located between the bladder and the rectum. It is composed of four parts – fundus, corpus (or body), cervix and internal os. The area of the body above the insertion of the fallopian tubes is called the fundus. The inner thin echogenic layer of the uterus is called the endometrium and the outer muscular layer is called the myometrium. The normal thickness of the endometrium in the post-menopausal woman is less than 5 mm.

3.14 MRA of the abdominal aorta

A Superior mesenteric artery.
B Gastroduodenal artery.
C Common hepatic artery.
D Splenic artery.
E Left internal iliac artery.

The branches of the aorta can be recognized by the position from which they arise off the aorta:

Branch	Artery
Anterior	Coeliac trunk
	Superior mesenteric artery
	Inferior mesenteric artery
Lateral	Inferior phrenic
	Middle suprarenal
	Renal
	Gonadal
Posterior	Lumbar
	Median sacral

The coeliac trunk is the first major branch of the aorta and gives rise to three arteries:

Splenic artery	Takes a horizontal tortuous course to the left
Left gastric artery	Takes a vertical course and is not seen on this image as it overlies the aorta
Common hepatic artery	Courses to the right

The gastroduodenal artery takes a vertical inferior course and arises from the proximal common hepatic artery.

3.15 Axial CT of the abdomen with IV contrast

A Fissure of the falciform ligament.
B Lateral limb of right adrenal gland.
C Portal vein.
D Left diaphragmatic crus.
E Splenic artery.

The falciform ligament is a thin peritoneal fold that attaches the left lobe of the liver to the peritoneum of the anterior abdominal wall. The adrenal glands are retroperitoneal structures that lie superior to the kidneys and are found at the level of T12/L1. They are not visualized on routine ultrasound in adults but can be seen in neonates. CT and MRI are the best forms of imaging for the glands. They are composed of a body and a medial and lateral limb.

3.16 Axial CTA of the lower limbs

A   Right tibialis anterior muscle.
B   Right short saphenous vein.
C   Left posterior tibial artery.
D   Left peroneal artery.
E   Left anterior tibial artery.

The tibialis anterior can be easily located as it is the largest muscle of the anterior compartment of the leg, running lateral to the tibia. The short saphenous vein can be readily identified as it is the only large vessel running subcutaneously along the posterior aspect of the leg. It arises from the lateral aspect of the dorsal venous arch, passes posterior to the lateral malleolus and drains into the popliteal vein within the popliteal fossa. The popliteal artery bifurcates at the lower border of popliteus into the anterior tibial artery and the tibioperoneal trunk (which further divides into the posterior tibial artery and peroneal artery). The anterior tibial artery can be recognized on axial section as it runs in the anterior compartment of the lower limb. The posterior tibial artery can also be recognized as it passes posterior to the tibia as described in the name of the vessel. The peroneal artery runs medial to the fibula on axial section as demonstrated in the image.

3.17 Axial STIR MRI of the left ankle

A   Left tibialis anterior tendon.
B   Left extensor hallucis tendon.
C   Left flexor hallucis longus tendon.
D   Left flexor digitorum longus tendon.
E   Left tibialis posterior tendon.

The mnemonic for remembering the order of contents of the flexor retinaculum of the lower limb as it passes medial to the tibia is **T**om, **D**ick, **AN**d, **H**arry, which corresponds to **T**ibialis posterior, flexor **D**igitorum longus, posterior tibial **A**rtery, tibial **N**erve and flexor **H**allucis longus.

The soleus is one of the muscles of the posterior superficial compartment of the leg. On axial images of the ankle, the tibialis anterior is the most medial anterior tendon, as demonstrated. A mnemonic to remember the anterior tendons of the ankle joint from medial to lateral is **T**om **H**ates **D**ick, corresponding to **T**ibialis anterior, extensor **H**allucis longus and extensor **D**igitorum longus.

3.18 Axial CT of the abdomen with IV contrast

A   Linea alba.
B   Left rectus abdominis muscle.
C   Left internal oblique muscle.
D   Left external oblique muscle.
E   Left transversus abdominis muscle.

The rectus abdominis runs vertically down the centre of the abdomen and is divided in its midline by the linea alba. It is enclosed by the rectus sheath, which is formed by the aponeurosis of the external oblique, internal oblique and transversus abdominis (from anterior to posterior).

3.19 Axial T1 MRI of the right femur

A Rectus femoris muscle.
B Vastus intermedius muscle.
C Sartorius muscle.
D Gracilis muscle.
E Semitendinosus muscle.

There are four quadriceps muscles:

* Rectus femoris.
* Vastus medialis.
* Vastus intermedius.
* Vastus lateralis.

The rectus femoris can be recognized on axial section as the anterior muscle that lies directly in the midline. The sartorius is identified as the small superficial muscle overlying the superficial femoral vessels as it forms the roof of the adductor canal through which the vessels travel. The gracilis is recognized easily by its thin elongated shape and it is the most medial muscle of the thigh.

The semitendinosus is one of the hamstrings of the thigh. It originates from the ischial tuberosity and inserts into the upper medial surface of the tibia. To recognize the semitendinosus on axial section, remember that it is the smallest of the posterior muscles of the thigh, usually lies in the midline posterior to the femur and runs in between the biceps femoris (laterally) and the semimembranosus (medially).

When trying to differentiate semimembranosus from semitendinosus, remember semiTendinosus is laTeral to semimembranosus or semiMembranosus is Medial to semitendinosus.

For further images and descriptions of the thigh muscles see Questions 5.17, 6.19 and 7.20.

3.20 Longitudinal ultrasound of the right infant hip

A Ilium.
B Femoral capital epiphysis.
C Labrum.
D Acetabulum.
E Triradiate cartilage.

Ultrasound of the paediatric hip is used for detection and follow-up of developmental dysplasia of the hip. The infant is positioned in the lateral decubitus position with the hip flexed and the probe orientated longitudinally. As the femoral head is unossified it can be easily visualized resting within the bony acetabulum. It appears as a speckled circular hypoechoic structure in the centre of the image. Sometimes an ossification centre can be visualized in the femoral head but this is not demonstrated on this image. The iliac bone is seen as the straight line running from the left of the picture and should transect the femoral head. The labrum is seen as the hypoechoic rim of tissue running between the acetabulum and the femoral head.

Examination 4: Questions

Question 4.1

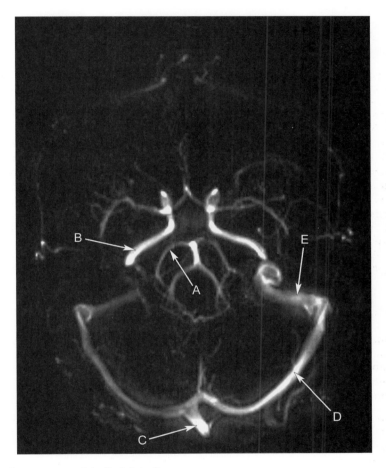

Name the structures labelled **A** to **E**.

Question 4.2

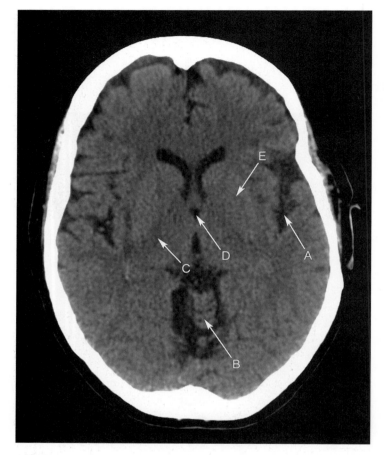

Name the structures labelled **A** to **E**.

Question 4.3

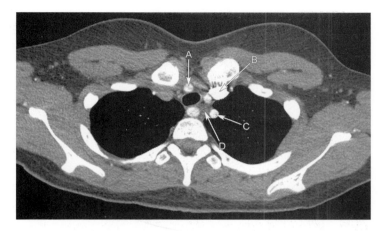

Name the structures labelled **A** to **D**.
E What normal variant is present?

Question 4.4

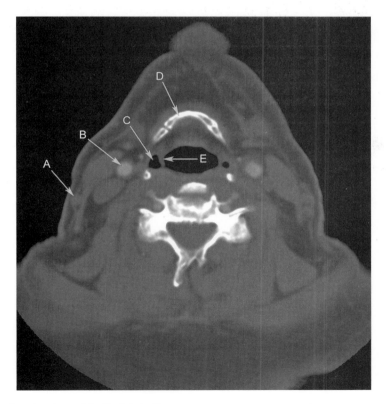

Name the structures labelled **A** to **E**.

Question 4.5

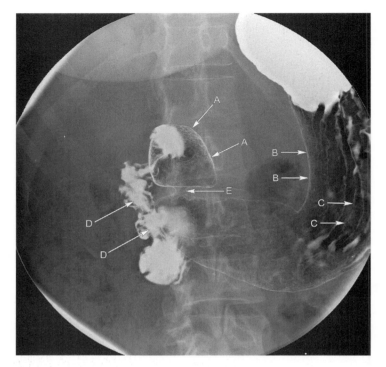

Name the structures labelled **A** to **E**.

Question 4.6

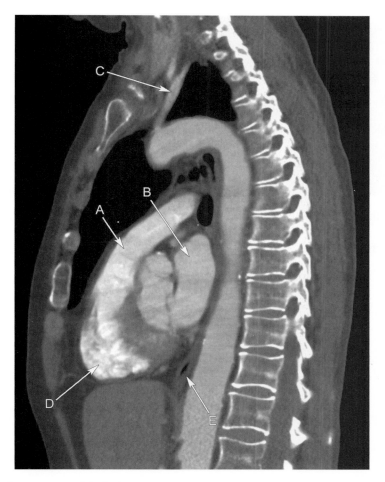

Name the structures labelled **A** to **E**.

Question 4.7

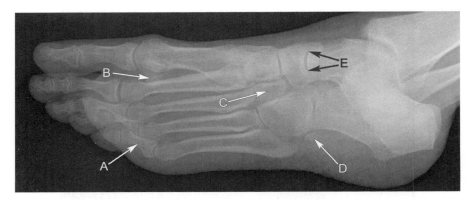

Name the structures labelled **A** to **E**.

Question 4.8

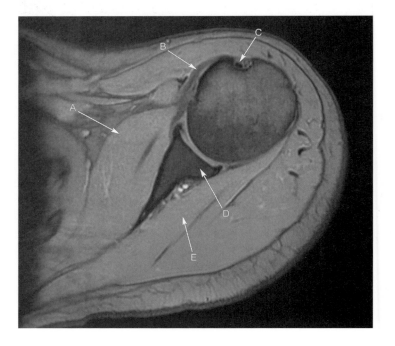

This is an axial MRI of the shoulder.
Name the structures labelled **A** to **E**.

Question 4.9

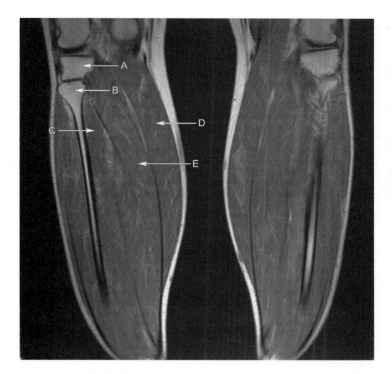

Name the structures labelled **A** to **E**.

Question 4.10

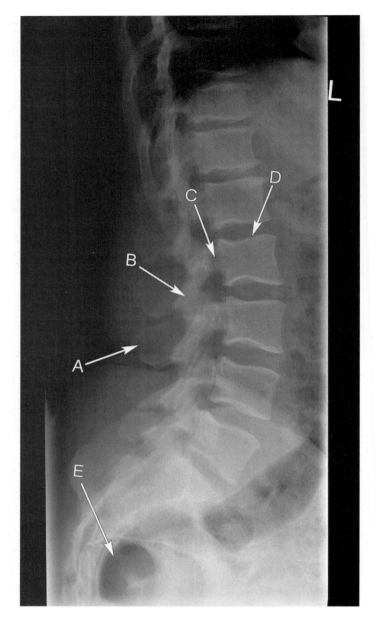

Name the structures labelled **A** to **E**.

Question 4.11

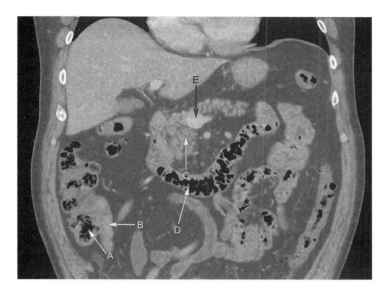

Name the structures labelled **A** to **E**.

Question 4.12

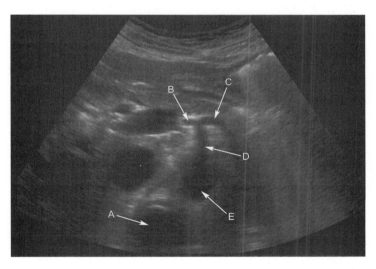

A What vertebral level is this?
Name the structures labelled **B** to **E**.

Question 4.13

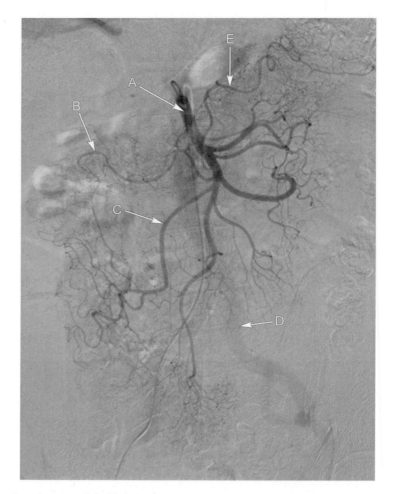

Name the structures labelled **A** to **E**.

Question 4.14

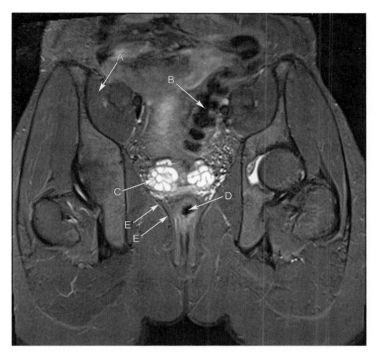

Name the structures labelled **A** to **E**.

Question 4.15

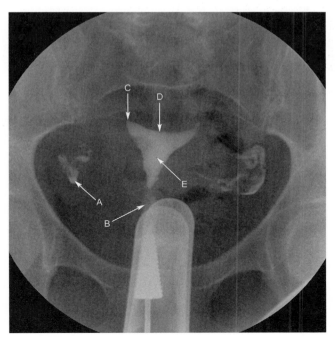

Name the structures labelled **A** to **E**.

Question 4.16

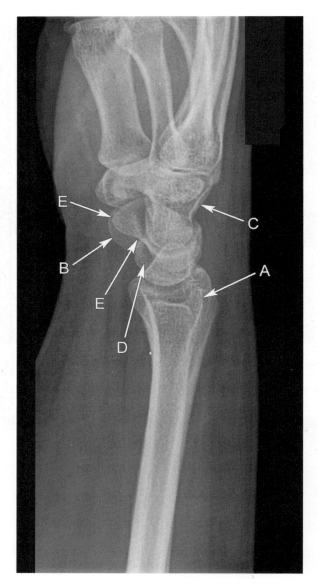

Name the structures labelled **A** to **E**.

Question 4.17

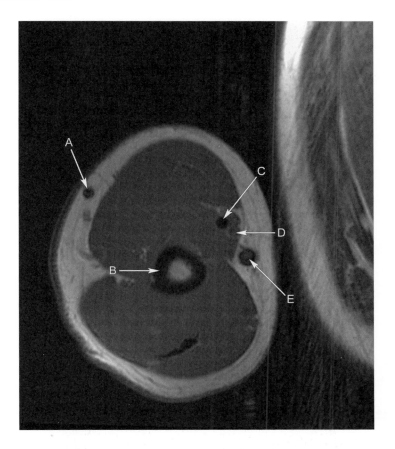

This is an axial MR through the upper arm.
Name the structures labelled **A** to **E**.

Question 4.18

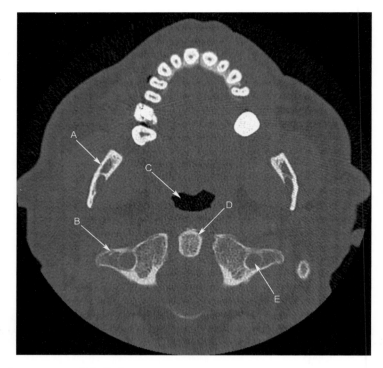

Name the structures labelled **A** to **E**.

Question 4.19

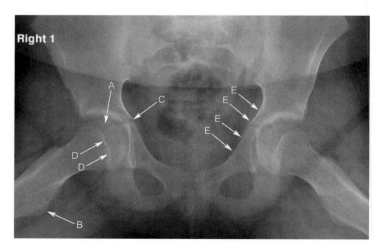

Name the structures labelled **A** to **E**.

Question 4.20

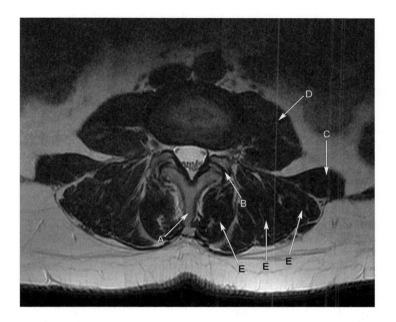

This is an axial MRI of the lumbar spine at the level of the L3/4 intervertebral disc. Name the structures labelled **A** to **E**.

Examination 4: Answers

4.1 MRV of the venous sinuses of the brain

A Right posterior cerebral artery.
B Right internal carotid artery.
C Superior sagittal sinus.
D Left transverse sinus.
E Left sigmoid sinus.

A diagram to aid remembering the sequence:

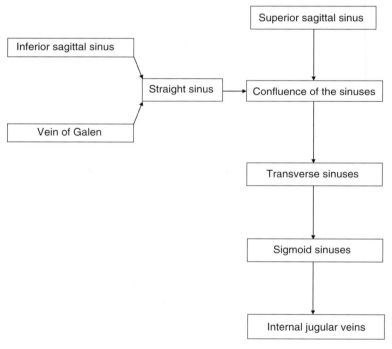

Figure 4.1 Sequence of venous sinuses of the brain

See Question 3.5 for a further description of the venous sinuses of the brain.

4.2 Axial CT of the brain

A Left sylvian fissure.
B Cerebellar vermis.
C Posterior limb of the right internal capsule.
D Third ventricle.
E Left lentiform nucleus.

On brain CT the white matter appears darker than the cortical grey matter. The internal and external capsules are white matter tracts and can therefore be visualized as low attenuation lines adjacent to the basal ganglia. The external capsule is lateral to the lentiform nucleus and medial to the insular cortex. Cerebrospinal fluid spaces within the brain can be readily identified by their fluid attenuation and appear almost black.

The ventricular system of the brain is continuous with the central canal of the spinal cord. There are four ventricles – the right and left lateral ventricles, the third ventricle and the fourth ventricle. The lateral ventricles are large C-shaped structures, which have frontal, temporal and occipital horns. The third ventricle lies within the midline between the thalami and the fourth ventricle which lies within the hindbrain. They all communicate via different foramina. The following flow diagram depicts the ventricular system and the foramina:

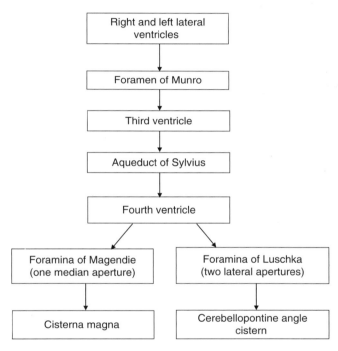

Figure 4.2 The ventricular system and the foramina

4.3 Axial CT of the chest with IV contrast

A Brachiocephalic artery.
B Left brachiocephalic vein.
C Left subclavian artery.
D Oesophagus.
E Aberrant right subclavian artery.

A left-sided aortic arch with an aberrant right subclavian artery is the most common congenital anomaly of the aortic arch. The aberrant right subclavian artery usually arises distal to the origin of the left subclavian, passes behind the oesophagus and anterior to the vertebral column in the superior mediastinum. The aberrant right subclavian may cause dysphagia due to external compression. This is termed dysphagia lusoria. A barium swallow classically demonstrates an oblique posterior extrinsic impression on the oesophagus with an inferior-to-superior (left-to-right) course.

See Question 5.13 for further discussion of the oesophageal impressions seen on barium swallow.

4.4 Axial CT of the neck with IV contrast

A Right external jugular vein.
B Right common carotid artery.
C Right piriform fossa.
D Hyoid bone.
E Right aryepiglottic fold.

The external jugular vein is formed within the parotid gland by the junction of the retromandibular vein and the posterior auricular vein. The vessel courses down within the superficial tissues along the posterior border of the sternocleidomastoid to drain into the subclavian vein. The right common carotid artery is a branch of the brachiocephalic artery, whereas the left common carotid artery is a direct branch of the aortic arch.

The aryepiglottic folds arise from the inferolateral aspect of the epiglottis and insert into the arytenoid cartilages. They define the piriform fossae laterally with the vestibule of the larynx medially.

4.5 Double contrast barium meal

A Duodenal cap.
B Lesser curve.
C Gastric folds (rugae).
D Second part of the duodenum.
E Pylorus.

The mucosal lining of the stomach has tiny nodular elevations called areae gastricae (they can be seen in the antrum of the stomach on this image), which are within expandable folds called the gastric rugae. The gastric rugae increase the surface area of the stomach; this increases absorption as well as providing the ability for the stomach to expand and contract with meals. The gastric rugae are usually 3–5 mm thick.

The duodenum is composed of four parts, generally referred to as D1, D2, D3 and D4. The first part (D1) includes the duodenal cap, which is well demonstrated in this image. It is a smooth-walled structure located immediately after the pylorus, and is the only part of the duodenum that is intraperitoneal. The remainder of the first part of the duodenum is retroperitoneal and ends at the superior duodenal flexure. The second part of the duodenum (D2) commences at the superior duodenal flexure and takes a vertical course to the inferior duodenal flexure where the third part of the duodenum (D3) starts. The pancreatic and common bile ducts enter the second part of the duodenum via the ampulla of Vater.

4.6 Sagittal CT chest with IV contrast

A Pulmonary trunk.
B Left atrium.
C Left subclavian artery.
D Right ventricle.
E Oesophagus.

The pulmonary trunk arises from the right ventricle, lies anterior to the aorta and passes posteriorly and inferiorly to the arch of the aorta where it bifurcates into the left and right pulmonary arteries.

There are openings in the diaphragm to allow the passage of structures between the thorax and abdomen. The three major openings and their corresponding vertebral levels are:

Vertebral level	Structure
T8	Inferior vena cava Right phrenic nerve
T10	Oesophagus Vagus nerve Oesophageal branches of the left gastric artery
T12	Aorta Azygos and hemiazygos vein Thoracic duct

The vertebral levels are easy to remember as they are multiples of two starting from eight. And the number of structures in each can be recalled as the 2–3-3 formation.

4.7 AP oblique X-ray of the left foot

A Proximal phalynx little (fifth) left toe,
B Left sesamoid bone.
C Left lateral cuneiform.
D Left os peroneum.
E Left talonavicular joint.

There are a number of accessory ossicles of the foot, which are normal variants and should not be confused with fractures. The os peroneum is an accessory ossicle located lateral to the cuboid.

A sesamoid bone is a bone embedded in a tendon, the largest example in the body being the patella (located within the quadriceps tendon). They are also found in the hand adjacent to the head of the first metacarpal (within the tendons flexor pollicis brevis and adductor pollicis). Within the foot, two sesamoid bones are located adjacent to the head of the first metatarsal (both within the tendon of flexor hallucis brevis).

Please refer to Question 1.20 for the other accessory ossicles of the foot and their locations.

4.8 Axial proton density MRI of the left shoulder

A Left subscapularis muscle.
B Left subscapularis tendon.
C Left biceps brachii tendon.
D Left glenoid.
E Left infraspinatus muscle.

Biceps brachii literally translated in Latin means 'two headed of the arm', meaning that the muscle is composed of two muscles with separate origins but which share a common insertion (the radial tuberosity). The short head of the biceps attaches to the coracoid process of the scapula whereas the long head travels, as demonstrated within this image, within the intertubercular groove of the humerus through the joint capsule to insert to the supraglenoid tubercle of the scapula.

A joint capsule is the envelope surrounding a synovial joint. The shoulder capsule completely surrounds the shoulder attaching around the glenoid of the scapula beyond the glenoid labrum (the cartilaginous layer). Laterally, the capsule attaches to the anatomical neck of the humerus.

4.9 Coronal T1 MRI of the lower limb

A Lateral right tibial plateau.
B Head of right fibula.
C Right tibialis posterior muscle.
D Right gastrocnemius muscle.
E Right soleus muscle.

Since the fibula runs posteriorly to the tibia it can be recognized that this coronal image is demonstrating the posterior compartment of the lower limb. The lateral relation of the fibula to the tibia also helps with orientation.

The gastrocnemius is the largest and most superficial muscle of the calf. It has two heads – medial and lateral. The medial head originates from the medial femoral condyle (seen in the top left corner of the image). The lateral head arises from the lateral femoral condyle. It then forms a common tendon with the soleus (the Achilles tendon) and inserts into the posterior surface of the calcaneum.

The soleus is also found within the superficial posterior compartment of the lower limb and is located just anterior to gastrocnemius. The tibialis posterior originates from the lateral surface of the tibia and the medial surface of the fibula and runs within the deep posterior compartment of the lower limb. Distally it passes posterior to the medial malleolus (see Question 3.16) and then divides with many insertions in the foot (the major tendon inserting into the tuberosity of the navicular). It can be readily identified as it is the most central of all the muscles of the lower limb.

To see lower limb musculature in axial section please refer to Question 9.16.

4.10 Lateral X-ray of the lumbar spine

A Spinous process of L3.
B Inferior articular facet of L2.
C Pedicle of L2.
D Superior endplate of L2.
E Rectum.

There are five lumbar vertebrae. The superior and inferior margins of the vertebral bodies are termed the superior and inferior endplates. The intervertebral discs lie between the endplates of adjacent vertebrae and are not usually seen on X-rays. The lumbar spine (as demonstrated in this image) and cervical spine have a natural lordosis (or anterior curvature). The thoracic spine has a natural kyphosis (or posterior curvature).

Each thoracic vertebra has paired pedicles that arise from the lateral surface of the vertebral body. These are difficult to separate on the lateral X-ray as the structures overlap. There are paired superior and inferior facets that allow articulation with the adjacent vertebra and are best visualized on the lateral projection. The spinous processes of the lumbar vertebrae are bigger, thicker and broader than their cervical and thoracic counterparts. They are also more square-shaped and angled horizontally, rather than the caudal angulation of the thoracic spinous processes. The transverse processes are not visualized owing to their horizontal orientation.

4.11 Coronal CT of the abdomen with IV contrast

A Caecum.
B Terminal ileum.
C Uncinate process of the pancreas.
D Third part of the duodenum.
E Porto-splenic confluence; origin of portal vein.

The portal vein is formed by the union of the superior mesenteric vein and the splenic vein behind the neck of the pancreas. The uncinate process of the pancreas arises from the inferior aspect of the head of the pancreas and passes inferiorly to the portal vein and posteriorly to the superior mesenteric vessels. The head of the pancreas lies within the concavity of the second part of the duodenum. The terminal ileum is the only site for vitamin B12 and bile absorption within bowel and is commonly affected by disease processes such as Crohn's disease and TB. It enters the caecum of the colon as demonstrated in this image.

4.12 Transverse ultrasound of the abdomen

A T12.
B Common hepatic artery.
C Splenic artery.
D Coeliac trunk or axis.
E Aorta.

Radiologists should be comfortable assessing the aorta with ultrasound as it is part of a routine abdominal ultrasound. The aorta and the inferior vena cava can be identified as the two vessels running down the midline anterior to the vertebrae, with the aorta on the patient's left. The coeliac trunk is the first major branch of the abdominal aorta and arises off the aorta at the vertebral level of T12. It can be seen in the transverse plane as a short trunk anteriorly in the midline before dividing into a 'Y'. The fork on the patient's left is the splenic artery and the fork on the right is the common hepatic artery. This classic ultrasound view is called the 'seagull' sign.

4.13 Superior mesenteric angiogram

A Superior mesenteric artery.
B Right colic artery.
C Ileocolic artery.
D Left common iliac artery.
E Middle colic artery.

The superior mesenteric artery (SMA) is an anterior midline branch of the abdominal aorta arising at the level of L1, approximately 1 cm inferior to the coeliac trunk. It passes posteriorly to the neck of the pancreas and anteriorly to the uncinate process, travelling to the left of the superior mesenteric vein. The superior mesenteric artery supplies part of the pancreas and the small bowel from the distal duodenum to the distal two-thirds of the transverse colon. The ascending colon can be faintly recognized on the right of the image, thus allowing identification of the colonic branches of the superior mesenteric artery.

The branches of the superior mesenteric artery are listed in the following table:

Small bowel branches	Inferior pancreaticoduodenal artery	Distal duodenum Head of the pancreas
	Intestinal branches	Jejunum Ileum
Colonic branches	Ileocolic artery	Ileum Caecum and appendix Ascending colon
	Right colic artery	Ascending colon
	Middle colic artery	Transverse colon to the distal two thirds

4.14 Coronal T2 spin-echo MRI of the male pelvis

A Right iliacus.
B Sigmoid colon.
C Right seminal vesicle.
D Rectum.
E Right levator ani.

The seminal vesicles are paired structures that lie superiorly to the prostate and between the bladder and the rectum. Their function is to produce fluid that contributes to the ejaculate as it travels through the vas deferens. This fluid exits the seminal vesicles via the excretory ducts into the vas deferens as it enters the prostate gland. The seminal vesicles have a characteristic lobulated shape and their fluid content makes them readily identifiable on T2 weighted imaging.

4.15 Hysterosalpingogram (HSG)

A Ampulla of right fallopian tube (ampulla of right uterine tube).
B Cervix.
C Right uterine cornu.
D Fundus of uterus.
E Body of uterus.

The hysterosalpingogram is principally indicated for the investigation of infertility. It is typically performed in the fluoroscopy room, where contrast dye is injected into the uterus and a series of X-rays obtained. The aim is to identify any anatomical anomalies or obstruction to the fallopian tubes.

There are three radio-opaque structures at the base of this image. The two almost overlapping long structures are the vaginal speculum and the central structure is the metal cannula for introducing the dye.

The uterus consists of a cervix that extends into a body. The fundus lies opposite the cervix and in between the fallopian tubes. The uterine cornu are the two horns found one in each corner of the uterus in the superolateral extremity of the uterine body and mark the entrance for the fallopian tubes.

The fallopian tubes are about 10 cm long and lie within the broad ligament. They allow the passage of eggs from the ovary to the uterus. The fallopian tubes can be divided into four segments:

Infundibulum	The terminal part of the tube that terminates in the ostium and is surrounded by the fimbriae
Ampulla	Forms the major middle segment of the fallopian tube
Isthmus	The narrow segment that lies just lateral to the uterus
Intramural (interstitial)	The part of the tube that pierces the uterine wall to open into the uterine cavity

4.16 Lateral X-ray of the right wrist

A Right ulnar styloid.
B Right pisiform.
C Right capitate.
D Right lunate.
E Right scaphoid.

Assessing the alignment of the carpal bones on a lateral X-ray is common every-day practice in radiology. Remember the 'order of the cups and cap'. The lunate sits within the cup of the radius and the capitate sits within the cup of the lunate, i.e. radius **CUP** lunate **CUP CAP**itate.

If there is loss of the alignment of this column of cups then a lunate or perilunate dislocation should be suspected. Indeed the pathognomonic sign of a lunate disloca-tion is the 'spilled tea cup' sign, where the 'cup' (lunate) is seen to point or 'spill' onto the palm.

When assessing the lateral wrist X-ray for trauma, it is important to assess the angle between the scaphoid and the lunate to detect scapholunate dissociation.

4.17 Axial T1 MRI of the right arm

A Right cephalic vein.
B Right humerus.
C Right brachial vein.
D Right brachial artery.
E Right basilic vein.

The cephalic and basilic veins are superficial veins of the arm. The cephalic vein commences on the radial side of the dorsal venous network on the hand and ascends along the radial border of the arm. The cephalic vein then courses along the lateral border of the biceps before piercing the coracoclavicular fascia to drain into the axil-lary vein. The basilic vein commences on the ulnar side of the dorsal venous network and ascends up the medial border of the biceps brachii of the upper arm before con-tinuing as the axillary vein at the lower border of the teres major. The brachial vein is a deep vein of the arm and travels alongside the brachial artery before joining the axillary vein at the lower border of the subscapularis.

4.18 Axial CT of the cervical spine

A Right mandible.
B Right transverse process of atlas (C1).
C Nasopharynx
D Dens; odontoid peg
E Left foramen transversarium

C1 is known as the atlas bone and forms the joint between the skull and the spine. It is unique as it has no body. It is ring-shaped and consists of an anterior and posterior arch with two lateral masses. Each lateral mass has a superior and inferior articular facet. C2 is known as the axis. There is no intervertebral disc between C1 and C2.

The pharynx conducts food to the digestive tract and air to the lungs and extends from the base of the skull to the level of the cricoid cartilage or C6 (where the larynx and oesophagus commence). It is split into the nasopharynx, oropharynx and hypopharynx (or laryngopharynx).

Nasopharynx	Lies posterior to the nose and extends from the skull base to the level of the soft palate (~C2)
Oropharynx	Extends from the soft palate to the level of the hyoid bone (C3)
Hypopharynx or laryngopharynx	Extends from the level of the hyoid bone to the level of the cricoid cartilage (C6)

4.19 Frog-leg X-ray of the pelvis

A Right femoral capital epiphysis.
B Right lesser trochanter.
C Right triradiate cartilage or 'Y' cartilage of the acetabulum.
D Right femoral capital epiphyseal plate or physis.
E Left iliopectineal line.

The frog-leg lateral pelvis X-ray is taken with the child supine with the knees flexed and the legs abducted with the heels together. It is used for the child presenting with hip pain for detection of a slipped capital femoral epiphysis. The femoral epiphysis first slips posteriorly before moving medially. This is why the subtle posterior movement of the epiphysis is best viewed on the lateral projection. The triradiate cartilage is the common physis of the three pelvis bones (the ilium, ischium and pubis), from which acetabular growth occurs.

4.20 Axial T2 MRI of the lumbar spine

A Spinous process of L3.
B Left L3/4 facet joint.
C Left quadratus lumborum muscle.
D Left psoas major muscle.
E Left erector spinae muscle.

The ligamentum flavum is a ligament that connects the laminae of the vertebrae and extends from C2 to S1. Hypertrophy of the ligamentum flavum is a factor that contributes to spinal stenosis, along with facet joint hypertrophy, osteophyte formation and bulging discs. The quadratus lumborum can be recognized as it lies laterally and posteriorly to the psoas and adjacent to the transverse processes. As the name suggests, it is quadrilateral in shape. It extends from the inferior surface of the 12th rib and inserts into the iliac crest.

The erector spinae is located either side of the spinous process of the vertebral column and is composed of three muscles, which can be remembered by the mnemonic 'I love spinach' (lateral to medial):

- Iliocostalis.
- Longissimus.
- Spinalis.

Examination 5: Questions

Question 5.1

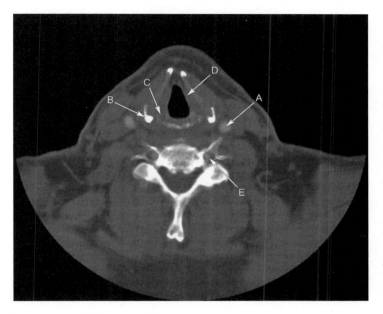

Name the structures labelled **A** to **E**.

Question 5.2

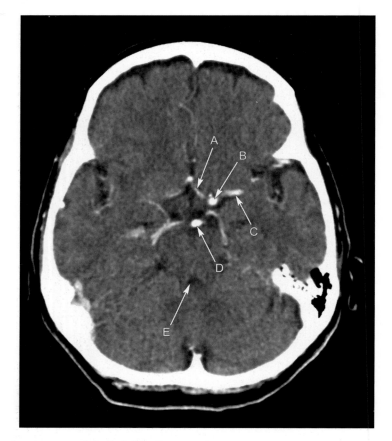

Name the structures labelled **A** to **E**.

Question 5.3

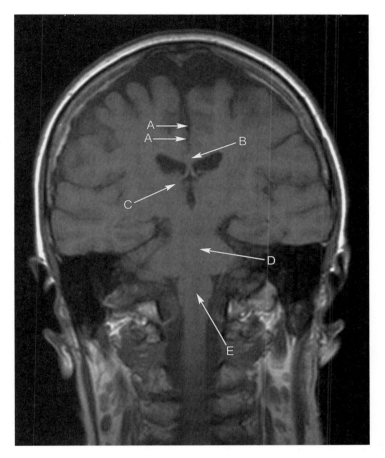

Name the structures labelled **A** to **E**.

Question 5.4

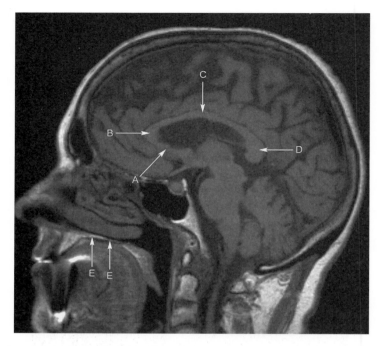

Name the structures labelled **A** to **E**.

Question 5.5

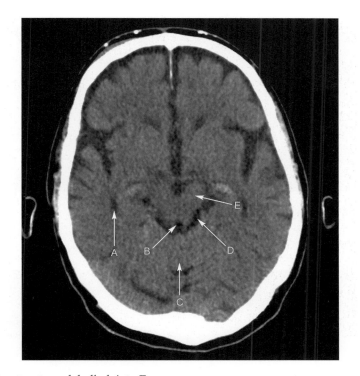

Name the structures labelled **A** to **E**.

Question 5.6

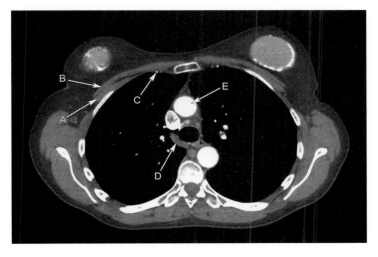

Name the structures labelled **A** to **E**.

Question 5.7

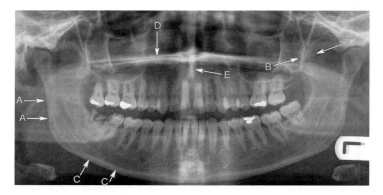

Name the structures labelled **A** to **E**.

Question 5.8

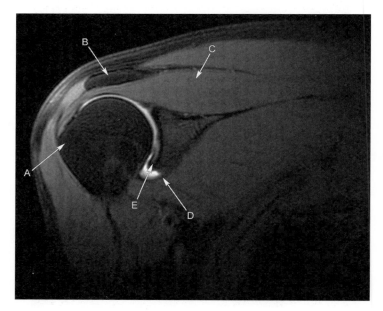

Name the structures labelled **A** to **E**.

Question 5.9

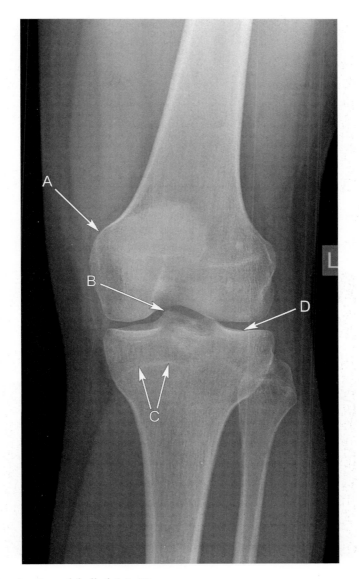

Name the structures labelled **A** to **D**.
E What structure attaches to **A**?

Question 5.10

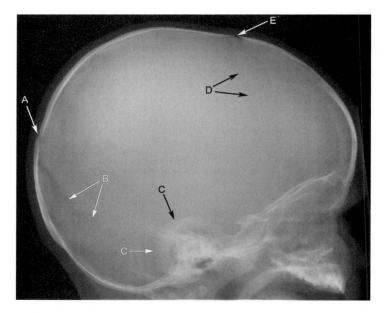

Name the structures labelled **A** to **E**.

Question 5.11

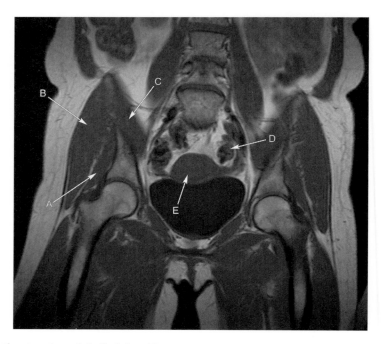

Name the structures labelled **A** to **E**.

Question 5.12

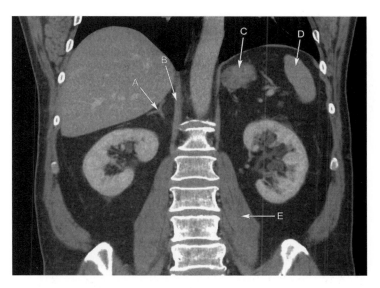

Name the structures labelled **A** to **E**.

Question 5.13

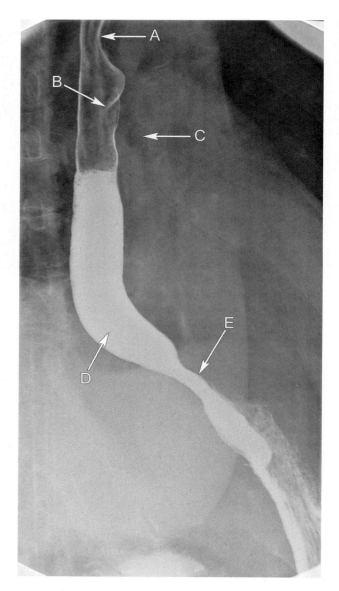

A What structure makes this impression?
B What structure makes this impression?
Name the structures labelled **C** to **E**.

Question 5.14

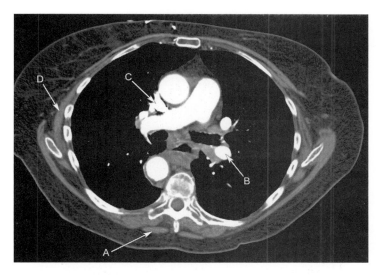

Name the structures labelled **A** to **D**.
E What normal variant is present?

Question 5.15

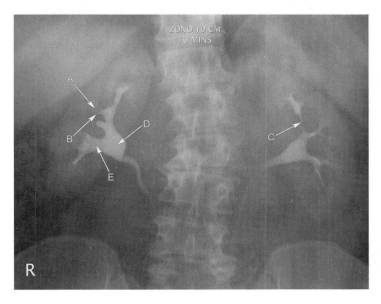

Name the structures labelled **A** to **E**.

Question 5.16

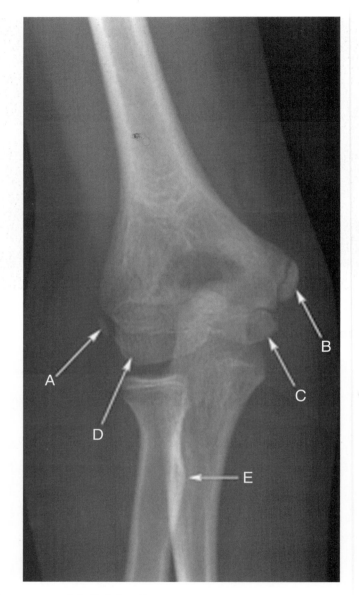

Name the structures labelled **A** to **E**.

Question 5.17

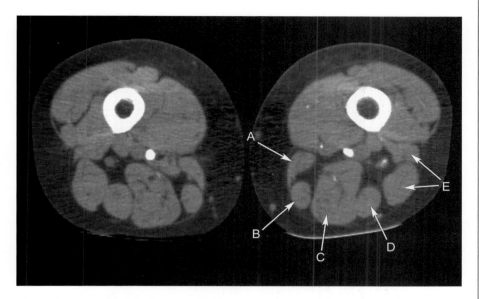

Name the structures labelled **A** to **E**.

Question 5.18

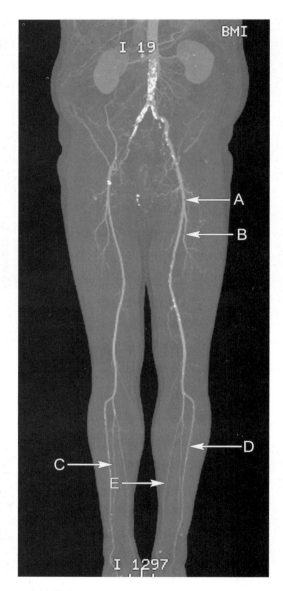

Name the structures labelled **A** to **E**.

Question 5.19

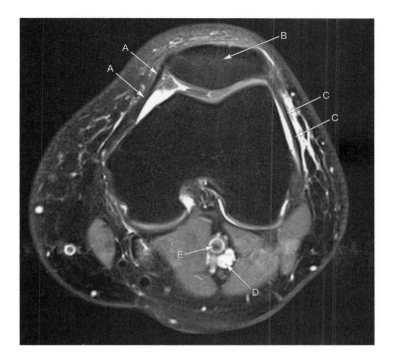

This is an axial MRI of the left knee.
Name the structures labelled **A** to **E**.

Question 5.20

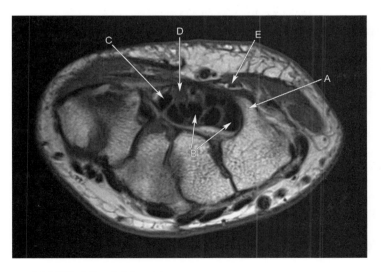

This is an axial MRI of the right wrist.
Name the structures labelled **A** to **D**.
E What structures pass through **E**?

Examination 5: Answers

5.1 Axial CT of the neck with IV contrast

A Left common carotid.
B Right thyroid cartilage.
C Right arytenoid cartilage.
D Left vocal cord.
E Left vertebral artery.

The larynx connects the hypopharynx to the trachea and contains the vocal cords, which are responsible for phonation. It is supported by a number of cartilaginous structures, including the cricoid, arytenoid and thyroid cartilages. The larynx is split into three subsites – the supraglottis, glottis and subglottis.

Supraglottis	Superior boundary is the tip of the epiglottis Inferior border is the laryngeal ventricle, which separates the false from the true vocal cords Contents include the epiglottis, false vocal cords, aryepiglottic folds and arytenoid cartilage
Glottis (pictured here)	At the level of the true vocal cords Contains the true vocal cords and the anterior and posterior commissure
Subglottis	Upper boundary is the inferior border of the true vocal cords Lower boundary is the inferior border of the cricoid cartilage or the first tracheal ring

5.2 Axial CT of the brain with IV contrast

A Left anterior cerebral artery.
B Left internal carotid artery.
C Left middle cerebral artery.
D Basilar artery tip.
E Aqueduct of Sylvius.

The circle of Willis is a circle of arteries that supplies the brain and includes:

- The anterior cerebral arteries.
- The anterior communicating artery.
- The internal carotid arteries.
- The posterior communicating arteries.
- The posterior cerebral arteries.

5.3 Coronal T1 MRI of the brain

A Interhemispheric fissure.
B Body of the corpus callosum.
C Right thalamus.
D Pons.
E Medulla.

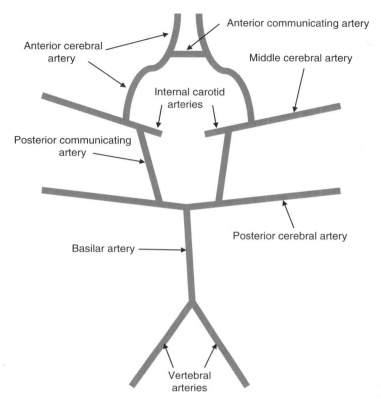

Figure 5.1 The circle of Willis

The coronal T1 sequence is part of the standard imaging protocol for MRI assessment of the brain. The interhemispheric fissure separates the two hemispheres of the brain. The falx cerebri is the arched fold of dura mater that runs vertically within the interhemispheric fissure. The thalami are paired midline structures that lie on either side of the third ventricle. When viewed in sagittal section (Question 5.4) the middle of the body of the corpus callosum can be seen to lie over the line of the brainstem.

5.4 Sagittal T1 MRI of the brain

A Rostrum of the corpus callosum.
B Genu of the corpus callosum.
C Body of the corpus callosum.
D Splenium of the corpus callosum.
E Hard palate.

The corpus callosum is the largest white matter structure of the brain. It connects the cerebral hemispheres of the brain and allows communication between them.

The corpus callosum is divided into five parts:

Genu	Anterior portion of the corpus callosum Genu is Latin for knee: this part can be seen to resemble a bent knee
Splenium	Posterior part of the corpus callosum PoSterior for Splenium
Body	Lies between the genu and the splenium

Isthmus	Thin posterior part between the body and the splenium
Rostrum	Rostrum is Latin for rooster: the rostrum is supposed to resemble the crest on a rooster
	Extends inferiorly and posteriorly from the genu

5.5 Axial CT of the brain

A Temporal horn of right lateral ventricle.
B Aqueduct of Sylvius.
C Cerebellar vermis.
D Quadrigeminal cistern.
E Midbrain.

The midbrain can be recognized by its characteristic shape and central concavity, whereas the pons has a convex anterior surface (see Question 6.1). Vermis is Latin for 'worm', and is used to describe the median narrow wormlike structure that connects the two cerebellar hemispheres. The quadrigeminal cistern is a cerebrospinal fluid filled space and extends laterally from the quadrageminal cistern around the midbrain of the brainstem to connect the interpeduncular cistern. The aqueduct of Sylvius connects the third ventricle to the fourth ventricle.

For further information on the cisterns of the brain see Question 2.5.

5.6 Axial CT chest with IV contrast

A Right pectoralis minor muscle.
B Right pectoralis major muscle.
C Right internal thoracic artery.
D Azygos vein.
E Ascending thoracic aorta.

The pectoralis major is the largest most anterior muscle of the anterior chest wall, underneath which lies the smaller pectoralis minor. The internal thoracic artery is one of the three branches of the first part of the subclavian artery (the other two being the thyrocervical trunk and the vertebral artery). It descends on the posterior surface of the anterior thorax lateral to the sternum, running deep to the internal intercostal muscles (and superficial to the transverse thoracic muscles). It divides at the sixth intercostal space into the musculophrenic artery and the superior epigastric artery (which continues the same inferior vertical course as the internal thoracic artery).

The azygos vein starts anterior to the L2 vertebra (variable), passes through the aortic hiatus and ascends along the posterior mediastinum to the right of the vertebral column. It provides venous return from the posterior thorax and abdomen to the superior vena cava. From T12–T5 the azygos vein travels anterior to the vertebral bodies and to the right of the aorta (as demonstrated in this image). At the level of T4, it arches anteriorly over the right main bronchus at the root of the right lung to drain into the superior vena cava.

5.7 Orthopantomogram (OPG)

A Right ramus of mandible.
B Coronoid process of left mandible.
C Body of right mandible.
D Hard palate.
E Nasal septum.

The OPG is a panoramic dental X-ray view of the upper and lower jaw displaying the upper and lower teeth and includes the temporomandibular joints on either side. The nature of the panoramic view demonstrates the hard palate as a straight line. The hyoid bone can also be seen in the bottom corners of the image. The mandible is made up of two halves, each half consisting of a body, an angle, a ramus, a coronoid process and a condylar neck and process.

5.8 Coronal MR arthrogram of the right shoulder

A Right greater tuberosity of the humerus.
B Right acromion.
C Right supraspinatus muscle.
D Right joint capsule.
E Right inferior glenoid labrum.

The supraspinatus initiates abduction of the shoulder and originates from the supraspinatus fossa of the scapula. This image demonstrates its passage immediately inferior to the acromion and its insertion onto the greater tubercle of the humerus. The space between the humeral head and the acromion is called the subacromial space; when it is narrowed the tendon of the supraspinatus is at risk of a tear. Of the rotator cuff muscles, the supraspinatus is most commonly torn (with its insertion at the greater tuberosity being the most common location). The inferior glenoid labrum is another important review area landmark when assessing shoulder MRI. The anterior inferior glenoid labrum is susceptible to injury following anterior shoulder dislocation (termed a Bankart lesion). This is often accompanied by a fracture of the posterior humeral head (termed a Hill–Sachs lesion).

5.9 AP X-ray of the left knee

A Left adductor tubercle.
B Left medial tibial spine.
C Left fused growth plate, proximal tibia.
D Left lateral tibial plateau.
E Left adductor magnus muscle.

A tubercle is a small protuberance of a bone. At the most superior aspect of the medial epicondyle of the femur is a small tubercle called the adductor tubercle. This is the insertion point for the adductor magnus. The tibial spine lies between the articular facets of the tibia. Fractures of the tibial spine (or the intercondylar eminence, as it otherwise known) can be subtle on radiographs of the knee and are associated with cruciate ligament injury. The area around the head of the fibula is another area that needs to be studied on trauma knee radiographs to look for the subtle Segond fracture (avulsion fracture of the lateral tibial condyle). Segond fractures have a high association with tears of the anterior cruciate ligament and injury to the medial meniscus.

5.10 Lateral X-ray of an infant's skull

A Posterior fontanelle.
B Lambdoid suture.
C Pinna.
D Coronal suture.
E Anterior fontanelle.

The coronal suture separates the parietal and frontal bones and can be recognized by its orientation in the coronal plane. The lambdoid suture derives its name from the shape of the Greek letter lambda (Λ). It is a posterior suture that separates the parietal, temporal and occipital bones. Knowledge of the sutures of the skull is essential for a radiologist, to help in differentiating between sutures and fractures on skull radiographs. Skull fractures usually appear as dark linear lines and are not usually located in anatomical areas, whereas skull sutures are located in anatomical areas and do not run in straight lines (as can be seen on this image).

The anterior fontanelle is located at the junction of the coronal and sagittal sutures and can take up to two years to close. The posterior fontanelle is located at the junction of the lambdoid and sagittal sutures and usually closes by the age of six months.

5.11 Coronal T1 MRI of the pelvis

A Right gluteus minimus muscle.
B Right gluteus medius muscle.
C Right iliacus muscle.
D Left ovary.
E Uterus.

The buttocks are made up of three gluteal muscles – gluteus maximus, gluteus medius and gluteus minimus. These muscles act as extensors and abductors of the hip joint. The gluteus maximus is the largest and most powerful of these, and its distal attachments are to the iliotibial band and gluteal tuberosity of the femur. It is innervated by the inferior gluteal nerve (L5, S1 and S2). The gluteus medius and minimus are innervated by the superior gluteal nerve (L5 and S1).

5.12 Coronal CT of the abdomen with contrast

A Right adrenal gland.
B Right diaphragmatic crus.
C Stomach.
D Spleen.
E Left psoas major muscle.

There are three main paired muscles in the posterior abdominal wall – psoas major, quadratus lumborum and iliacus. The psoas major runs from the sides of the T12–L5 vertebrae (including transverse processes and discs) to the lesser trochanter of the femur, where it joins with the psoas minor and iliacus to act as a flexor of the hip. This confluence of muscles is generally known as iliopsoas.

5.13 Barium swallow

A Impression of the arch of the aorta.
B Impression of the left main bronchus.
C Left main bronchus.
D Distal oesophagus.
E Gastro-oesophageal junction.

There are two normal indentations in the anterior and lateral aspect of the thoracic oesophagus. The most superior is the impression of the aortic arch, which often becomes more prominent with age. Just distal to this is the indentation caused by the left main bronchus. In 10% of patients the left inferior pulmonary vein causes an anterior indentation about 5 cm below the carina. Other extrinsic compressions on the thoracic aorta can indicate the presence of anatomical variants and abnormalities. Examples of these include a right-sided or double aortic arch, an aberrant subclavian artery and vascular rings.

- **Right-sided aortic arch**: right oesophageal impression, absent normal left arch impression.
- **Double aortic arch**: impression on the right and left side of the oesophagus, slightly higher and larger on the right. Described as characteristic 'reverse S-shaped indentation'.
- **Aberrant right subclavian artery**: posterior oesophageal indentation, obliquely upward to the right on AP views (see Question 4.3).
- **Aberrant left pulmonary artery**: anterior oesophageal impression.

5.14 Axial CT of the chest with IV contrast

A Right trapezius muscle.
B Left interlobar pulmonary artery.
C Superior vena cava.
D Right serratus anterior muscle.
E Right-sided descending thoracic aorta.

The trapezius muscle is a large superficial muscle of the back. There is one on each side, and taken together their shape resembles a trapezium. It has origins in the spinous processes of C7–T12 vertebrae and inserts into the lateral aspect of the clavicle and scapula. Its primary motor innervation is the accessory nerve (CN XI).

The image illustrates a right-sided descending thoracic aorta. This is a relatively common anomaly and is generally secondary to a right-sided aortic arch (although there are rare cases of a left-sided aortic arch with a right-sided descending thoracic aorta (circumflex aorta)).

There are several types of right-sided aortic arch, of which the most common are:

- **Type I**: mirror image (the great vessels originate in the normal order); 95% association with congenital cardiac abnormality.
- **Type II**: right-sided arch with aberrant left subclavian; 5–15% association with congenital cardiac abnormality.

5.15 Intravenous urogram

A Right upper pole papilla.
B Right upper pole fornix.
C Left upper pole infundibulum.
D Right renal pelvis.
E Right lower pole major calyx.

The renal collecting system is divided into three major calyces, each of which is subdivided into two or three minor calyces. Each minor calyx meets the apex of a renal pyramid, which is known as the renal papilla. The fornix is the acutely angled portion of the calyx alongside the papilla. The infundibulum is the funnel-shaped channel that connects the calyces to the renal pelvis, which in turn tapers to become the proximal ureter.

5.16 AP X-ray of the right elbow (paediatric)

A Right lateral epicondyle apophysis.
B Right medial epicondyle apophysis.

C Right trochlea epiphysis.
D Right capitellum epiphysis.
E Right radial tuberosity.

The order of appearance of the elbow ossification centres can be remembered by the mnemonic **CRITOL:**

- **C**apitellum (six months).
- **R**adial head (five years).
- **I**nternal (medial) epicondyle (seven years).
- **T**rochlea (nine years).
- **O**lecranon (eleven years).
- **L**ateral epicondyle (thirteen years).

The capitellum, trochlea and radial head contribute to longitudinal bone growth and make up an articular surface; they are therefore considered to be epiphyses. All of the other ossification centres of the elbow are apophyses.

5.17 Axial CT of the thigh with IV contrast

A Left sartorius muscle.
B Left gracilis muscle.
C Left semimembranosus muscle.
D Left semitendinosus muscle.
E Left biceps femoris muscle.

The thigh is divided into three facial compartments that are each supplied by a specific nerve:

Anterior compartment	Femoral nerve
Medial compartment	Obturator nerve
Posterior compartment	Sciatic nerve

The muscles in the posterior aspect of the thigh are known as the hamstrings, which consist of semitendinosus, semimembranosus and biceps femoris. These muscles span both the thigh and hip joint and are therefore both hip extensors and knee flexors. The anterior compartment contains the quadriceps muscle group and sartorius. The medial compartment contains the gracilis and the adductor muscle group.

5.18 Coronal CT angiogram of the lower limbs

A Left common femoral artery.
B Left profunda femoris artery.
C Right peroneal artery.
D Left anterior tibial artery.
E Left posterior tibial artery.

The anatomical landmark for the common femoral artery is the femoral head. The femoral artery divides into the superficial femoral artery and profunda femoris around 4 cm inferior to the inguinal ligament. The superficial femoral artery follows a relatively vertical course as compared with the femur, which is more oblique. It gives off no major branches in the thigh, a fact that can help distinguish it from the profunda femoris artery, which has six major branches (medial and lateral circumflex femoral arteries, along with four perforating arteries).

The three major arteries of the lower limb are the anterior tibial artery, the posterior tibial artery and the peroneal artery. The popliteal artery divides into the anterior and posterior tibial arteries at the level of the proximal tibiofibular joint. The posterior tibial artery then gives rise to the peroneal artery branch.

5.19 Axial PD MRI of the left knee

A Medial retinaculum.
B Patella.
C Lateral retinaculum.
D Popliteal vein.
E Popliteal artery.

The strong fibrous tissue planes found on the medial and lateral sides of the patella are known as the medial retinaculum and lateral retinaculum, respectively. They act to stabilize the patella during flexion and extension. The lateral retinaculum is an extension of the fibrous aponeurosis of the vastus lateralis muscle. The medial retinaculum is an extension of the fibrous aponeurosis of the vastus medialis muscle.

The popliteal artery is a continuation of the superficial femoral artery and lies deep to the popliteal vein.

5.20 Axial T1 MRI of the right wrist

A Hook of the right hamate.
B Tendons of right flexor digitorum profundus.
C Tendon of right flexor pollicis longus.
D Right median nerve.
E Right ulnar nerve and artery (the structure labelled is Guyon's canal).

The carpal tunnel is the fibro-osseous pathway on the palmar side of the wrist that connects the distal forearm to the deep palm. It is superficially bounded by the flexor retinaculum, which attaches medially to the pisiform and the hook of the hamate bone, and laterally to the scaphoid and trapezium. The carpal tunnel is a tight space containing ten structures in total:

- Nine flexor tendons.
- Four × flexor digitorum profundus.
- Four × flexor digitorum superficialis.
- Flexor pollicis longus.
- Median nerve.

Within the carpal tunnel, the median nerve lies superficially with respect to the tendons.

The ulnar nerve and artery pass through a separate channel, known as Guyon's canal.

Examination 6: Questions

Question 6.1

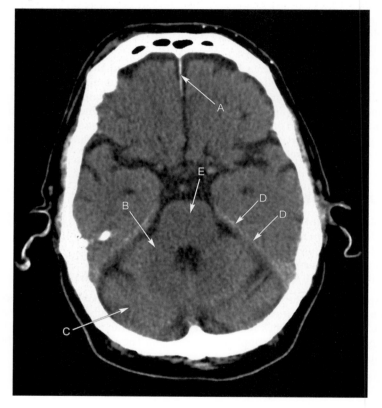

Name the structures labelled **A** to **E**.

Question 6.2

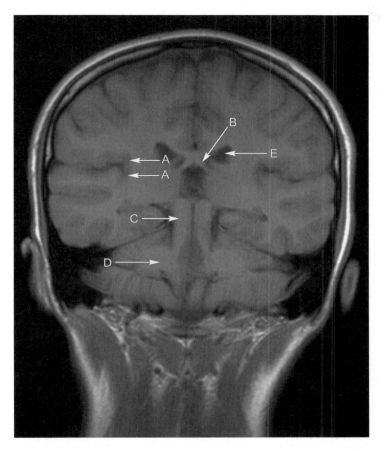

Name the structures labelled **A** to **E**.

Question 6.3

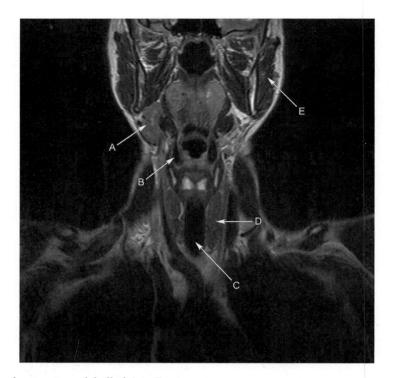

Name the structures labelled **A** to **E**.

Question 6.4

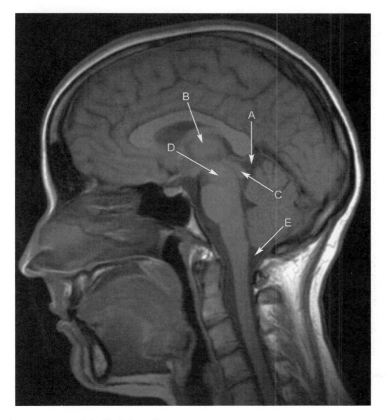

Name the structures labelled **A** to **E**.

Question 6.5

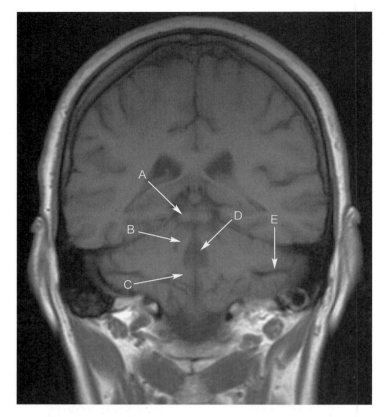

Name the structures labelled **A** to **E**.

Question 6.6

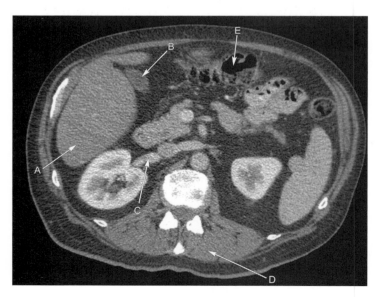

Name the structures labelled **A** to **E**.

Question 6.7

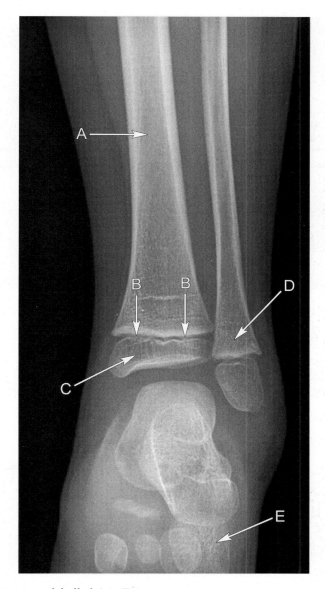

Name the structures labelled **A** to **E**.

Question 6.8

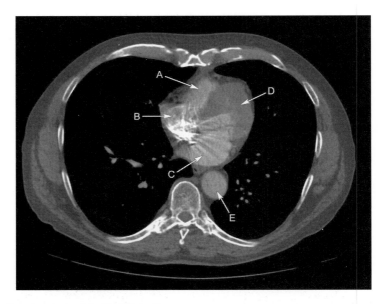

Name the structures labelled **A** to **E**.

Question 6.9

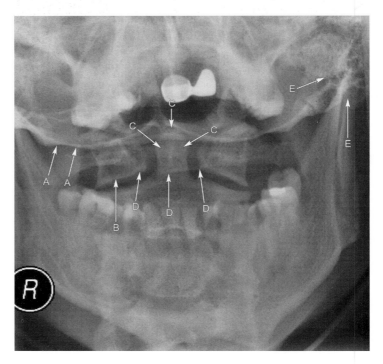

Name the structures labelled **A** to **E**.

Question 6.10

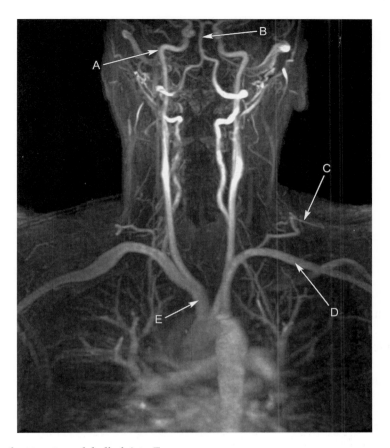

Name the structures labelled **A** to **E**.

Question 6.11

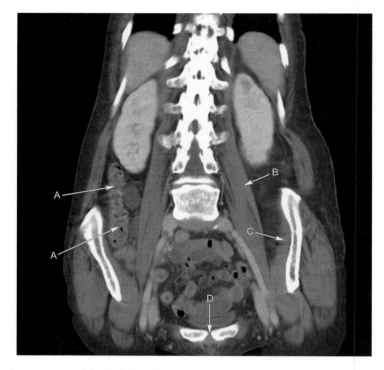

Name the structures labelled **A** to **D**.
E Which artery or arteries supply the structure labelled **A**?

Question 6.12

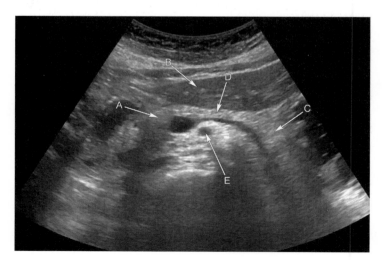

Name the structures labelled **A** to **E**.

Question 6.13

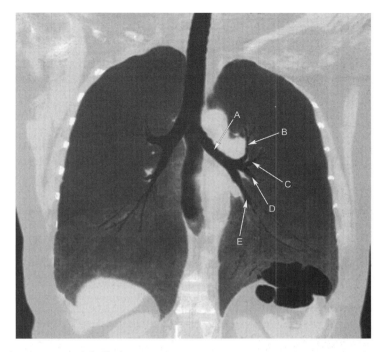

Name the structures labelled **A** to **E**.

Question 6.14

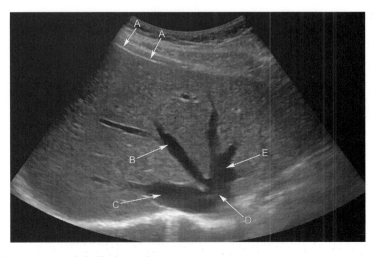

Name the structures labelled **A** to **E**.

Question 6.15

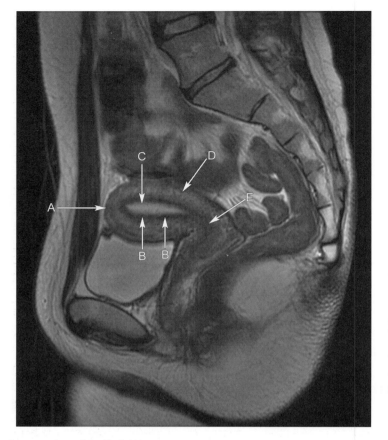

Name the structures labelled **A** to **E**.

Question 6.16

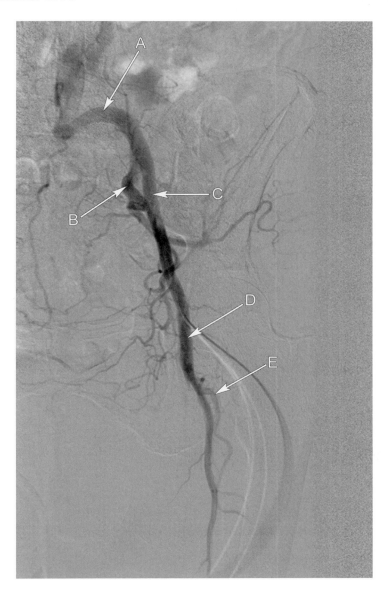

Name the structures labelled **A** to **E**.

Question 6.17

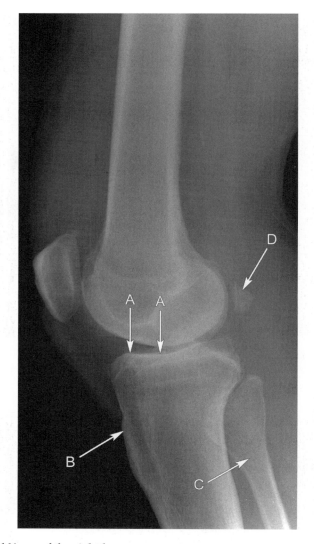

This is lateral X-ray of the right knee.
Name the structures labelled **A** to **D**.
E What structure may be damaged by a fracture at the level of **C**?

Question 6.18

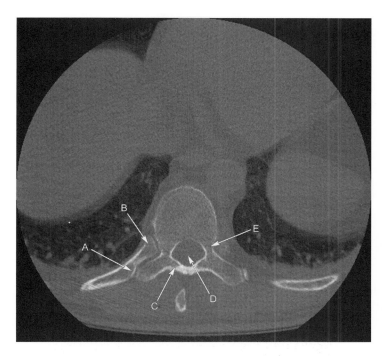

Name the structures labelled **A** to **E**.

Question 6.19

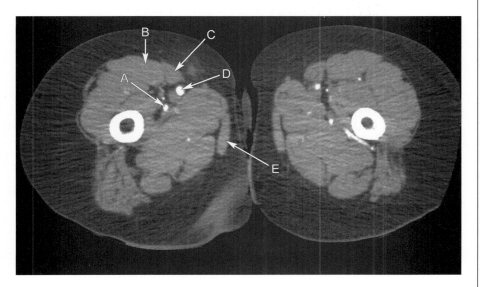

Name the structures labelled **A** to **E**.

Question 6.20

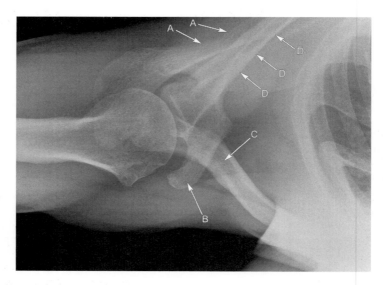

Name the structures labelled **A** to **D**.

E Which three muscles attach to the structure labelled **B**?

Examination 6: Answers

6.1 Axial CT of the brain

A Falx cerebri.
B Right middle cerebellar peduncle.
C Right cerebellar hemisphere.
D Left tentorium cerebelli.
E Pons.

The falx cerebri is a scythe-shaped fold of dura mater in the longitudinal fissure between the two cerebral hemispheres. It attaches anteriorly to the crista galli of the ethmoid and posteriorly to the upper surface of the tentorium cerebelli. The tentorium cerebelli is a tent of dura that separates the cerebellum from the inferior portion of the occipital lobe, thus defining the supratentorial and infratentorial spaces.

The cerebellum is connected to the rest of the central nervous system by three pairs of nerve tracts known as cerebellar peduncles. The inferior cerebellar peduncles connect the medulla spinalis and medulla oblongata with the cerebellum. They form a thick strand between the lower part of the fourth ventricle and the roots of the ninth and tenth cranial nerves. The middle cerebellar peduncles connect the pontine nuclei to the contralateral cerebellum. Their fibres are arranged in three fasciculi – superior, inferior and deep. The superior cerebellar peduncles connect the cerebellum to the midbrain. They form the upper lateral boundaries of the fourth ventricle. The anterior medullary velum connects the superior cerebellar peduncles, and between them they also form the roof the fourth ventricle.

6.2 Coronal T1 MRI of the brain

A Right insula.
B Left fornix.
C Midbrain.
D Right middle cerebellar peduncle.
E Left lateral ventricle.

The insula is an area of pronounced grey-white differentiation readily seen on CT and MRI. It is located between the sylvian fissure and external capsule, and is supplied by small perforating branches of the middle cerebral artery. Loss of the insular stripe is an early sign of middle cerebral artery (MCA) territory stroke. The fornix is a C-shaped bundle of white matter fibres that connects the hippocampus to the mammillary bodies and septal nuclei. The fibres at the hippocampus are known as the fimbria. The separate left and right sides are known as the crus of the fornix, and where they come together in the midline is called the body of the fornix.

6.3 Coronal T1 MRI of the neck

A Right submandibular gland.
B Right piriform fossa.
C Trachea.
D Left lobe of the thyroid.
E Left masseter muscle.

The submandibular glands lie in the floor of the mouth anterior to the angle of the mandible and superior to the digastric muscles. Each submandibular gland is divided into superficial and deep lobes, which are separated by the mylohyoid muscle. The piriform fossae are recesses on either side of the larynx and a common site for food trapping. They are bounded medially by the aryepiglottic fold and laterally by the thyroid cartilage and hyothyroid membrane. The masseter is a muscle of mastication running from the zygomatic process and arch to the mandible.

6.4 Sagittal T1 MRI of the brain

A Quadrigeminal cistern.
B Massa intermedia.
C Tectum (quadrigeminal plate).
D Midbrain.
E Cisterna magna.

The thalami form the majority of the lateral walls of the third ventricle. In 70–80% of people there is a midline interthalamic adhesion known as the massa intermedia. It is made up of nerve cell bodies and a few nerve fibres. The exact function of this adhesion is not known and its absence does not cause any functional defects.

The cerebellum is also well demonstrated on this image. It is divided into two hemispheres, which are then further subdivided by the deep fissures into lobules. The primary fissure (fissura prima) defines the anterior cerebellar lobe from the posterior lobe.

It is worth having a general understanding of the blood supply to the cerebellum. There are three main arteries that supply it:

Superior cerebellar artery (SCA – branch of the distal basilar artery)	Superior surface of the cerebellar hemispheres down to the horizontal fissures Superior vermis Dentate nucleus Majority of the cerebellar white matter
Anterior inferior cerebellar artery (AICA – branch of the proximal basilar artery)	Middle cerebellar peduncle Flocculus Antero-inferior surface of the cerebellum
Posterior inferior cerebellar artery (PICA – branch of the distal vertebral arteries)	Postero-inferior cerebellar hemispheres to the horizontal fissure Inferior vermis

6.5 Coronal T1 MRI of the brain

A Right inferior colliculus.
B Right superior cerebellar peduncle.
C Right inferior cerebellar peduncle.
D Fourth ventricle.
E Left horizontal fissure of the cerebellum.

There are four colliculi located on the anterior half of the midbrain – two superior and two inferior. Together they form part of the corpora quadrigemina. The superior colliculi are above the trochlear nerve and are visual processing centres. The inferior colliculi are involved in auditory processing.

6.6 Axial CT of the abdomen with IV contrast

A Right lobe of the liver (segment VI).
B Gallbladder.
C Right renal vein.
D Left erector spinae muscle.
E Transverse colon.

The liver is traditionally divided into anatomical right and left lobes. These are demarcated on the anterior surface by the falciform ligament and on the posterior surface by the grooves for the ligamentum teres and ligamentum venosum. There are two further described lobes that are part of the right liver lobe – the quadrate lobe and caudate lobe. The quadrate lobe is situated anteroinferiorly between the gallbladder bed and the fissure for the ligamentum teres. The caudate lobe lies posteriorly between the inferior vena cava and the fissure for the ligamentum venosum. In addition to this anatomical classification, the liver is also described as consisting of eight functionally discrete segments. For further information about segmental anatomy of the liver, see Questions 8.19 and 10.5.

The gallbladder lies within the gallbladder fossa. The posterior surface is covered by visceral peritoneum and the anterior surface is adherent to the liver.

6.7 AP X-ray of a paediatric ankle

A Left tibial diaphysis.
B Left tibial physis (or epiphyseal plate).
C Left tibial epiphysis.
D Left fibular metaphysis.
E Left cuboid.

Long bones can be divided into three sections – the diaphysis (shaft), metaphysis (junction between diaphysis and epiphysis), and the epiphysis (expanded articular end of a long bone). In the paediatric skeleton the growth plate (physis) is seen in between the metaphysis and the epiphysis.

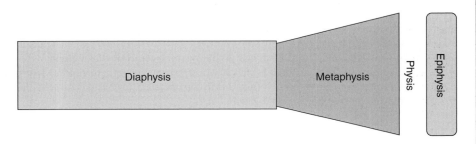

Figure 6.1 The paediatric skeleton

6.8 Axial CT of the chest with IV contrast

A Right ventricle.
B Right atrium.
C Left atrium.
D Left ventricle.
E Descending thoracic aorta.

Some tips to help identify the cardiac chambers:

- **Left atrium**: upper-posterior; square-shaped; smooth-walled; lies anterior to the oesophagus.
- **Right atrium**: right side of heart; right heart border on chest X-ray; anterior to left atrium.
- **Right ventricle**: anterior; triangular; lower part often touches lower part of sternum.
- **Left ventricle**: left side; thick walled; trabeculated; thickest chamber.

6.9 X-ray of the odontoid peg

A Occipital bone.
B Right lateral mass of C1.
C Odontoid peg.
D Anterior arch of C1.
E Left mastoid air cells.

The odontoid peg (dens) is a bony projection from the body of C2 (axis). The peg articulates with the posterior surface of the anterior arch of the atlas and has ligamentous attachments to the atlas and occipital bone. Fractures of the peg are classified into three different types:

Type I	Fracture through the tip
Type II	Fracture through the base (most common)
Type III	Fracture through the body of C2

6.10 Coronal MR angiogram of the neck

A Right internal carotid artery.
B Basilar artery.
C Left suprascapular artery.
D Left subclavian artery.
E Brachiocephalic artery.

The common carotid arteries bifurcate into the internal and external carotid arteries at approximately the C3 or C4 level. The internal carotid artery has no branches in the neck. The basilar artery supplies blood to the posterior part of the circle of Willis and arises from the confluence of the two vertebral arteries. The left subclavian artery is usually the third aortic arch branch (excluding the coronary arteries). The brachiocephalic artery is the first aortic arch branch.

6.11 Coronal CT of the abdomen with IV contrast

A Ascending colon.
B Left psoas major muscle.
C Left iliacus muscle.
D Symphysis pubis.
E Right colic artery and ileocolic artery.

The caecum is the first part of the large bowel and lies in the right iliac fossa. It does not have a mesentery. The terminal ileum enters it medially and obliquely, forming a valve known as the ileocaecal valve. The arterial supply of the caecum is the ileocolic artery (a branch of the superior mesenteric artery). The arterial supply of the ascending colon and hepatic flexure is via the ileocolic and right colic arteries.

6.12 Transverse ultrasound of the abdomen

A Head of pancreas
B Left lobe of the liver
C Tail of pancreas
D Body of pancreas
E Superior mesenteric artery

The pancreas lies transversely across the posterior abdominal wall behind the stomach and with the transverse mesocolon at its anterior margin. The head lies in the curve of the second part of the duodenum and gives rise to an uncinate process. The common bile duct passes posteriorly to the head of the pancreas. The neck of the pancreas is adjacent to the pylorus. The portal vein is formed posteriorly to the neck at the confluence of the splenic vein and superior mesenteric vein. The body of the pancreas curves across the midline and is closely related to the splenic vessels. The tail of the pancreas lies in the splenic hilum, within the splenorenal ligament.

6.13 Coronal CT of the chest

A Left main bronchus.
B Left upper-lobe bronchus.
C Superior segment of the lingular bronchus.
D Inferior segment of the lingular bronchus.
E Left lower-lobe bronchus.

The trachea divides into the left and right main bronchi. Each main bronchus then divides into secondary bronchi (lobar bronchi), of which there are two on the left and three on the right (left upper and lower lobe, right upper, middle and lower lobe). These secondary bronchi then subdivide into tertiary (segmental) bronchi that supply the bronchopulmonary segments, which are roughly pyramidal in shape.

There are three left upper-lobe bronchi (apical, posterior and anterior). The apical and posterior bronchi usually share a common apico-posterior bronchus prior to their division.

There are two lingular-lobe bronchi (superior segment and inferior segment). They arise from the left upper-lobe bronchus.

There are four left lower-lobe bronchi (apical, anterior, lateral and posterior). Unlike the right lower lobe, there is no medial basal bronchus.

For a table of the bronchial anatomy see Question 2.19.

6.14 Transverse ultrasound of the liver

A Liver capsule.
B Middle hepatic vein.
C Right hepatic vein.
D Inferior vena cava.
E Left hepatic vein.

The venous drainage of the liver is principally via the three hepatic veins – right, middle and left. These follow an intrahepatic course and typically join at the inferior vena cava. They are used as some of the landmarks for dividing the liver into segments.

It is important to assess the hepatic veins during routine liver ultrasound as their appearance and flow characteristics can be indicative of many disease processes. Engorgement of the hepatic veins and inferior vena cava can be a sign of right heart failure. Normal hepatic venous flow is pulsatile and triphasic like the jugular venous pulsation – alteration to this pattern can indicate hepatic venous thrombosis, which is suggestive of Budd–Chiari syndrome.

6.15 Sagittal T2 MRI of the female pelvis

A Fundus of uterus.
B Junctional zone.
C Endometrium.
D Myometrium.
E Cervix.

The uterus is an extra-peritoneal structure, lying between the bladder and the rectum. It can be divided into the fundus (the apex of the uterus), body and cervix. The endometrium is the lining of the uterine cavity and is seen as a hyperechoic stripe on ultrasound. The uterus is mostly smooth muscle that is known as myometrium, of which the innermost layer is the junctional zone. The junctional zone is an important structure to assess on imaging for endometrial carcinoma. It is best evaluated on T2-weighted MRI where it has a low signal compared than the myometrium. Tumours are considered to be confined to the endometrium when the junctional zone is preserved, although the junctional zone can be difficult to visualize in post-menopausal women.

6.16 Digital subtraction angiogram of the left leg

A Left common iliac artery.
B Left internal iliac artery.
C Left external iliac artery.
D Left common femoral artery.
E Left profunda femoris.

The aorta bifurcates into the left and right common iliac arteries at the level of L4. The common iliac artery runs along the medial side of the psoas muscles and bifurcates into internal and external branches at the level of L5/S1 (in front of the sacroiliac joint). The internal branch is the primary arterial supply of the pelvic organs and gluteal muscles. The external iliac artery continues along the medial border of the psoas and passes under the inguinal ligament. At the mid-inguinal point its name changes to the common femoral artery.

6.17 Lateral X-ray of the right knee

A Tibial plateau.
B Tibial tuberosity.
C Neck of fibula.
D Fabella.
E Common peroneal nerve.

The common peroneal nerve is a terminal division of the sciatic nerve. It passes obliquely along the lateral side of the popliteal fossa before wrapping around the head and neck of the fibula. Fractures of the fibula in this region can cause damage to the common peroneal nerve, leading to a foot drop.

The fabella is a sesamoid bone occasionally found within the tendon of the lateral head of gastrocnemius muscle. It is a normal variant present in approximately 10–30% of people and is frequently mistaken for a loose body. There can be two or three parts (fabella bipartita and tripartita). The tibial tuberosity gives rise to the patella ligament and is a common site of pathology in active adolescents (Osgood–Schlatter disease, also known as tibial tubercle apophyseal traction injury).

6.18 Axial CT of the thoracic spine

A Right articular tubercle of the rib.
B Right head of the rib.
C Right lamina.
D Vertebral canal/spinal cord.
E Left pedicle.

There are 12 thoracic vertebrae. The thoracic vertebrae have a smaller, more rounded vertebral canal than the cervical and lumbar vertebrae. T1–T10 vertebrae have facets for articulation with the tubercle of a rib. The pedicle is the segment between the transverse process and the vertebral body. The laminae are two broad plates, which extend dorsally and medially from the pedicles to fuse and complete the ring.

6.19 Axial CT angiogram of the thighs

A Right profunda femoris artery.
B Right rectus femoris muscle.
C Right sartorius muscle.
D Right superficial femoral artery.
E Right gracilis muscle.

The profunda femoris is the deep branch of the femoral artery, supplying blood to the medial and posterior compartments of the thigh as well as the hip joint. The rectus femoris is one of the quadriceps muscles. Superiorly it arises from the anterior inferior iliac spine and the ilium superior to the acetabulum. Inferiorly the quadriceps muscles unite to form the quadriceps tendon that attaches to the patella.

The sartorius muscle and gracilis muscle tendons unite with the semitendinosus muscle (so-called conjoined tendons) to form the pes anserinus on the medial aspect of the knee. This inserts into the anteromedial surface of the proximal tibia.

A mnemonic for the muscles of the conjoined tendon (medial to lateral) is 'Say Grace before Tea' (Sartorius, Gracilis, semiTendinosus).

6.20 Axial X-ray of the right shoulder

A Right spine of scapula.
B Right coracoid process.
C Right clavicle.
D Right scapula blade or body.
E Pectoralis minor, coracobrachialis and biceps brachii (short head).

The word coracoid is based on the Greek 'korax', which means 'raven's beak'. The coracoid process resembles this shape and is a small beak-like structure on the lateral edge of the antero-superior part of the scapula. The pectoralis minor muscle runs from the coracoid process to between the third and fifth ribs. The coracobrachialis muscle runs from the coracoid process to the medial side of the humeral shaft. The biceps brachii muscle runs from the coracoid process (short head) and the supra-glenoid tubercle (long head) to the radial tuberosity.

Examination 7: Questions

Question 7.1

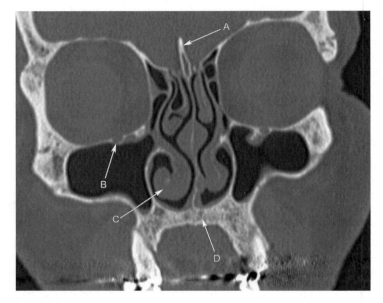

Name the structures labelled **A** to **D**.
E Name a structure that passes through **B**.

Question 7.2

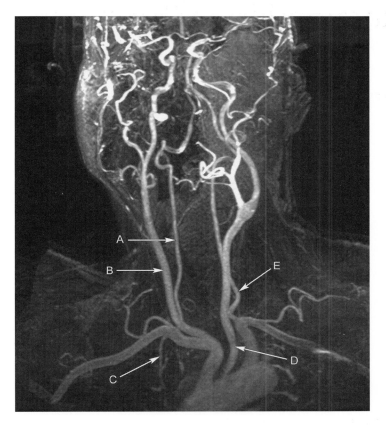

Name the structures labelled **A** to **E**.

Question 7.3

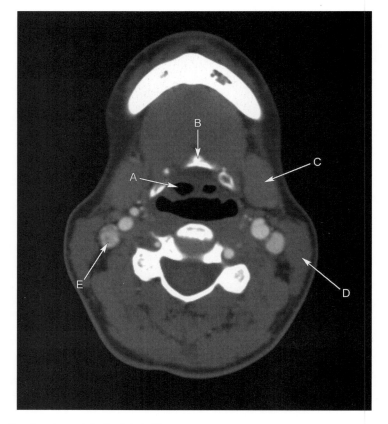

Name the structures labelled **A** to **E**.

Question 7.4

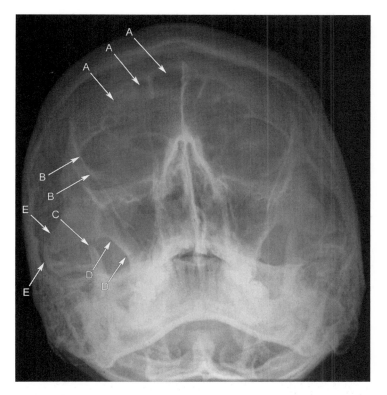

Name the structures labelled **A** to **E**.

Question 7.5

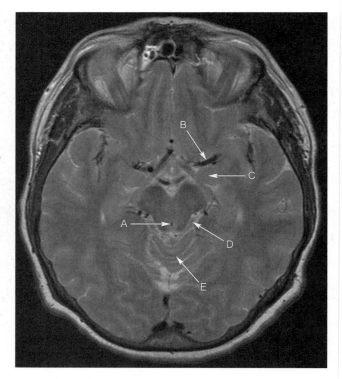

Name the structures labelled **A** to **E**.

Question 7.6

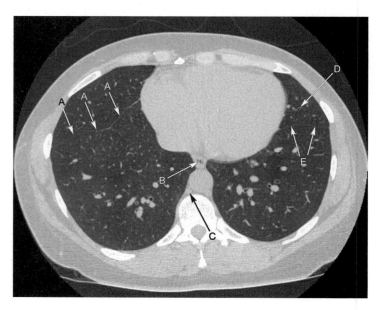

Name the structures labelled **A** to **E**.

Question 7.7

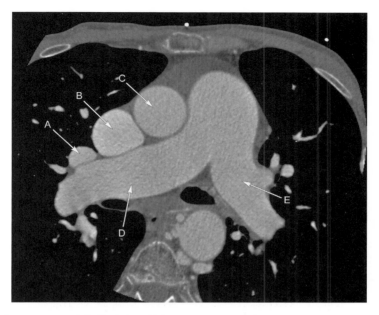

Name the structures labelled **A** to **E**.

Question 7.8

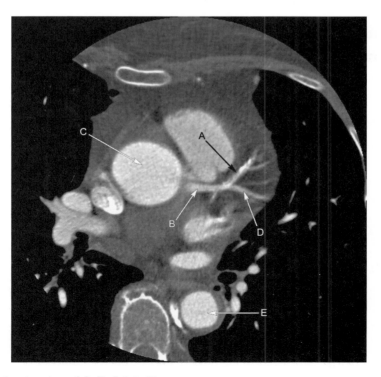

Name the structures labelled **A** to **E**.

Question 7.9

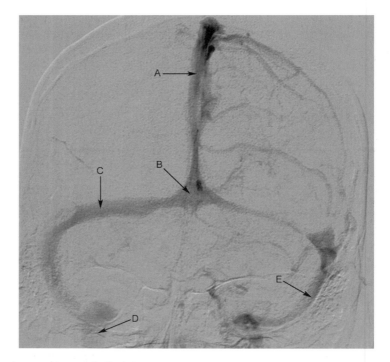

Name the structures labelled **A** to **E**.

Question 7.10

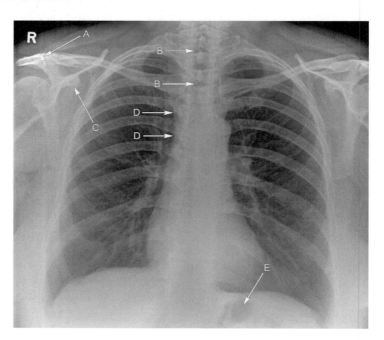

Name the structures labelled **A** to **E**.

Question 7.11

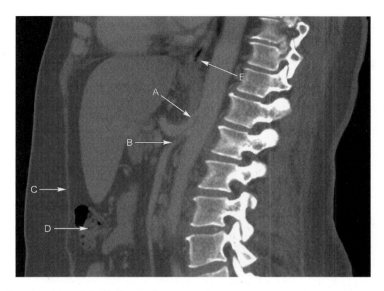

Name the structures labelled **A** to **E**.

Question 7.12

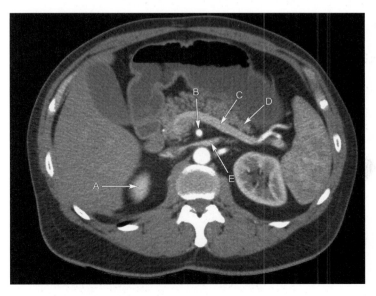

Name the structures labelled **A** to **E**.

Question 7.13

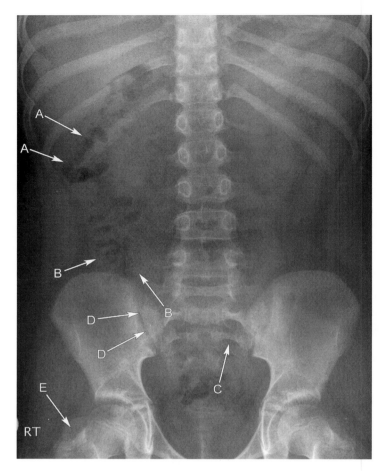

Name the structures labelled **A** to **E**.

Question 7.14

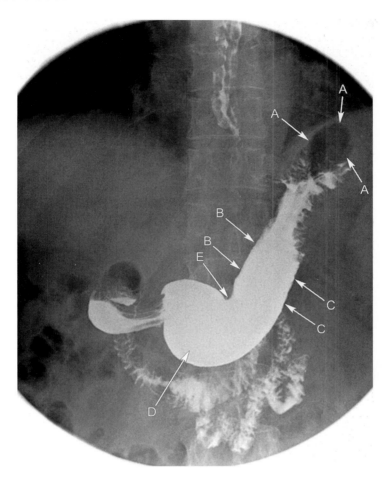

Name the structures labelled **A** to **E**.

Question 7.15

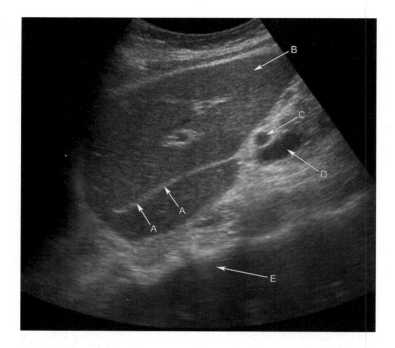

This is a longitudinal ultrasound through the abdomen.
Name the structures labelled **A** to **E**.

Question 7.16

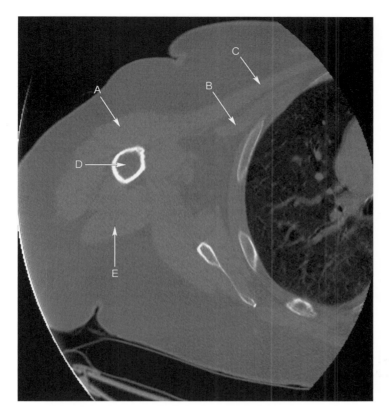

Name the structures labelled **A** to **E**.

Question 7.17

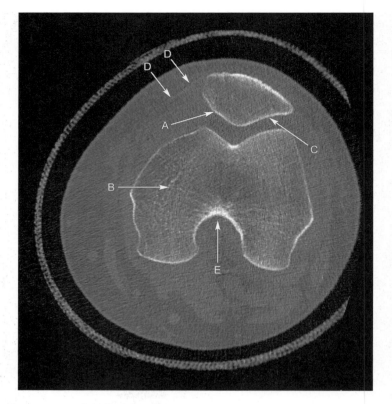

Name the structures labelled **A** to **E**.

Question 7.18

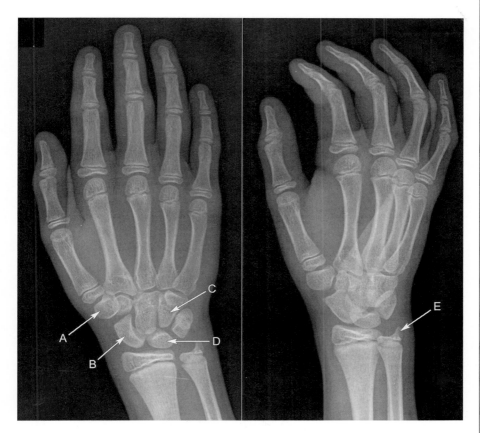

Name the structures labelled **A** to **E**.

Question 7.19

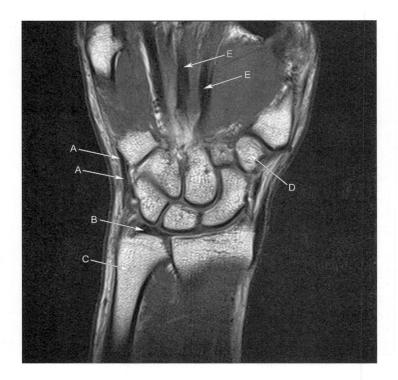

This is a coronal MRI of the left wrist.
Name the structures labelled **A** to **E**.

Question 7.20

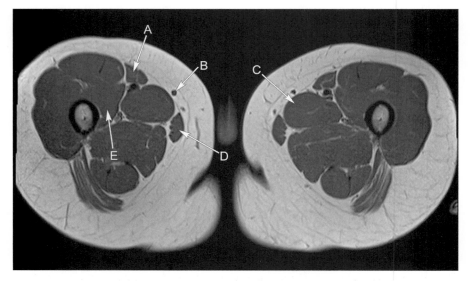

Name the structures labelled **A** to **E**.

Examination 7: Answers

7.1 Coronal CT of the sinuses

A Crista galli.
B Right infraorbital foramen.
C Right inferior turbinate.
D Hard palate.
E Right infraorbital nerve, artery or vein.

'Crista galli' is Latin for 'crest of the cock'. It is a midline ridge of bone that projects from the cribriform plate of the ethmoid bone. The falx cerebri attaches here, and the olfactory bulbs lie on either side. The infraorbital foramen transmits the infraorbital nerve, artery and vein, which can be damaged or compressed in orbital blowout fractures. The infraorbital nerve is a branch of the maxillary nerve, which is the second division of the trigeminal nerve (CN V).

There are three turbinates; superior, middle and inferior. They function to control the flow of air and ensure that even air humidification and warming takes place over an increased surface area. The osteomeatal complex is a functional entity that includes the middle turbinate, uncinate process, bulla ethmoidalis, hiatus semilunaris and ethmoid infundibulum. It is the common pathway for drainage and ventilation of the frontal, maxillary and ethmoid sinuses.

7.2 MR angiogram of the neck

A Right vertebral artery.
B Right common carotid artery.
C Right internal thoracic artery.
D Left common carotid artery.
E Left vertebral artery.

The paired vertebral arteries are branches of the first part of the subclavian arteries and course through the transverse foramen of each cervical vertebra from C6 to C1. After C1, the vertebral arteries pass through the suboccipital triangle and enter the foramen magnum. Within the skull they converge to form the basilar artery at the base of the medulla oblongata. The internal thoracic arteries originate from the subclavian arteries and supply the anterior chest wall and breasts. They divide into the musculophrenic and superior epigastric arteries at the level of the sixth rib.

7.3 Axial CT of the neck with IV contrast

A Right vallecula.
B Hyoid bone.
C Left submandibular gland.
D Left sternocleidomastoid muscle.
E Right internal jugular vein.

The valleculae (or valleculae epiglottica) are a pair of depressions on either side of the median glossoepiglottic fold. They are important landmarks during intubation and are the site where the laryngoscope blade is placed to help visualize the epiglottis.

The right internal jugular vein is one of a pair of vessels that form the major venous drainage of the brain and the superficial face and neck. It is formed in the jugular foramen from the confluence of the inferior petrosal sinus and the sigmoid sinus. It has a common trunk within the neck that drains the anterior branch of the retromandibular vein, facial vein, superior and middle thyroid veins, pharyngeal vein and lingual veins. The internal jugular veins descend in the carotid sheath and join the subclavian veins to form the brachiocephalic veins. The thoracic duct inlet typically lies at the junction of the left internal jugular vein and the left subclavian vein. For this reason, when siting subclavian central lines it is often recommended that the right subclavian vein is used instead of the left to minimize the risk of thoracic duct injury.

Further relevant images and descriptions of neck anatomy can be seen in Questions 4.4, 5.1 and 6.3.

7.4 X-ray of the face (Water's view)

A Frontal sinus.
B Greater wing of the right sphenoid bone (innominate line).
C Right coronoid process of the mandible.
D Lateral wall of the right maxillary sinus.
E Right zygomatic arch.

The frontal sinuses are absent at birth and generally only reach their full size at puberty. About 5% of people do not have a frontal sinus. The frontal sinuses connect to the middle meatus via the frontonasal duct. Their mucosal outline is innervated by the supraorbital nerve.

The maxilla forms the upper jaw, with the maxillary arch holding the upper teeth. It attaches laterally to the zygomatic bone. It helps form the roof of the mouth, the wall of the orbit and the lateral wall of the maxillary sinus.

The innominate line represents the tangentially viewed superior surface of the greater wing of the sphenoid bone (the squamo-zygomatic surface).

7.5 Axial T2 MRI of the brain

A Cerebral aqueduct (aqueduct of Sylvius).
B Left middle cerebral artery.
C Head of the left hippocampus.
D Ambient cistern.
E Cerebellar vermis.

The cerebral aqueduct (aqueduct of Sylvius) is a channel connecting the third and fourth ventricles. Blockage to this channel impedes the flow of cerebrospinal fluid and can cause hydrocephalus. The ambient cistern is an extension of the quadrigeminal cistern, extending laterally around the midbrain. It acts as a connection between the quadrigeminal cistern and the interpeduncular cistern. The cerebellar vermis lies in between the cerebellar hemispheres and is the site of termination of the spinocerebellar pathways.

7.6 Axial high resolution CT of the chest

A Right oblique fissure.
B Oesophagus.
C Azygos vein.
D Lingula of the left upper lobe.
E Left oblique fissure.

The right lung is divided into three lobes (upper, middle and lower) divided by two interlobar fissures. The right oblique fissure separates the right lower lobe from the right upper and middle lobes. The right horizontal fissure separates the right upper lobe from the right middle lobe. The left lung is divided into two main lobes (upper and lower), plus a lingular lobe (part of the left upper lobe). The left oblique fissure separates the left lower lobe from the left upper lobe. A knowledge and appreciation of the lung fissures is important when planning CT-guided lung biopsies. It is generally undesirable to insert the instrument into more than one lobe during a lung biopsy, therefore traversing fissures should be avoided where possible.

7.7 Axial cardiac CT with IV contrast

A Right superior pulmonary vein.
B Superior vena cava.
C Ascending aorta.
D Right main pulmonary artery.
E Left main pulmonary artery.

The pulmonary veins carry oxygenated blood from the lungs to the left atrium of the heart. They are notable in containing no valves. There are four main pulmonary veins – left superior, left inferior, right superior and right inferior. At the root of the lung the superior pulmonary vein lies anteroinferior to the pulmonary artery. The bronchus lies behind the pulmonary artery, as can be seen on this image.

The ascending aorta arises from the left ventricle at the level of the third costal cartilage just to the left of the sternum. At the highest point of its arch it reaches the level of the anterior margin of the second costal cartilage. In cases of chest paint or trauma it is important to assess the ascending aorta carefully for evidence of dissection.

7.8 Axial cardiac CT with IV contrast

A Left anterior descending artery.
B Left main coronary artery.
C Root of ascending aorta.
D Left circumflex artery.
E Descending thoracic aorta.

In general, there are two main coronary arteries – left and right. The left coronary artery arises from the left aortic sinus (left sinus of Valsalva) just above the aortic valve. It branches into the left anterior descending artery and the left circumflex artery. The left circumflex artery follows the left part of the coronary sulcus and gives rise to the marginal arteries. It supplies the posterolateral left ventricle and the sinoatrial node (in 40% of people). The left anterior descending artery passes along the anterior interventricular sulcus and typically supplies the anterolateral myocardium, apex, interventricular septum and around 50% of the left ventricle.

7.9 Cerebral venogram

A Superior sagittal sinus.
B Confluence of sinuses (torcular herophili).
C Right transverse sinus.
D Right internal jugular vein.
E Left sigmoid sinus.

There is a complex and highly variable network of cerebral cortical veins that drain into the dural sinus system. These veins run in superficial paths along the cortical sulci to drain the cerebral cortex and white matter. Owing to their variability and complexity, most of these veins are not named. There are a few important cerebral cortical veins that can be consistently identified on imaging. Their anatomy and dominance is, again, highly variable.

Superficial middle cerebral vein (or superficial sylvian vein)	Passes along the sylvian fissure and drains into the sphenoparietal sinus Connects with the vein of Labbé and the vein of Trolard
Vein of Labbé	Anastomotic vein Crosses the temporal lobe Connects the superficial middle cerebral vein to the transverse sinus
Vein of Trolard	Anastomotic vein Connects the superficial middle cerebral vein to the superior sagittal sinus

For further relevant images and explanation of the cerebral venous system, please see Questions 3.5 and 4.1.

7.10 X-ray of the chest

A Right acromioclavicular joint.
B Trachea.
C Right coracoid process.
D Superior vena cava.
E Stomach.

The acromioclavicular joint (AC joint) is a synovial joint connecting the scapula to the clavicle. It is stabilized by the superior and inferior acromioclavicular ligaments, and is a common site of sporting injuries. The normal acromioclavicular joint space is less than 5 mm. There is a further connection between the scapula and clavicle via the coracoclavicular ligament (which connects the coracoid process to the clavicle). The normal coracoclavicular distance is less than 12 mm. When assessing chest X-rays it is important also to inspect the shoulder joints, as it not uncommon to pick up unexpected pathology.

7.11 Sagittal CT of the abdomen with IV contrast

A Coeliac axis.
B Superior mesenteric artery.
C Linea alba.
D Transverse colon.
E Oesophagus.

There are three main anterior branches of the aorta supplying the abdominal viscera and bowel. These are the coeliac axis, superior mesenteric artery and the inferior mesenteric artery. The coeliac axis originates at T12 and gives rise to the common hepatic, left gastric and splenic arteries. The superior mesenteric artery arises at L1 and gives rise to the inferior pancreaticoduodenal artery, middle colic artery, right colic artery, intestinal arteries and the ileocolic artery. It typically runs to the left of the superior mesenteric vein – if it is seen to the right of the vein then suspect malrotation or volvulus.

The linea alba (white line) is the vertical midline aponeurosis of the anterior abdominal wall muscles.

For further images and explanations of the abdominal vasculature, see Questions 3.14, 6.11 and 10.18.

7.12 Axial CT of the abdomen with IV contrast

A Superior pole of the right kidney.
B Superior mesenteric artery.
C Splenic vein.
D Tail of pancreas.
E Left renal vein.

The superior mesenteric artery arises at L1 just below the coeliac axis. It supplies the pancreas and bowel from the distal duodenum to two-thirds of the transverse colon. The splenic vein is the primary venous drainage of the spleen and runs along the posterior surface of the pancreas. It joins with the superior mesenteric vein to become the portal vein at the porto-splenic confluence. The left renal vein is longer than the right renal vein, owing to the right-sided position of the inferior vena cava in relation to the aorta, and passes anterior to the aorta at the level of L1.

7.13 X-ray of the abdomen

A Hepatic flexure of colon.
B Caecum.
C Left S2 foramina.
D Right sacroiliac joint.
E Right greater trochanter.

The hepatic flexure is the bend of colon between the ascending colon and the transverse colon. It is supplied by the right colic artery (a branch of the superior mesenteric artery).

The sacroiliac (SI) joint is the largest axial joint in the body. Only the anterior third of the sacroiliac joint is a true synovial joint. The rest of the joint is composed of a complex set of fibro-ligamentous connections.

7.14 Barium follow-through

A Fundus.
B Lesser curve.
C Greater curve.
D Antrum.
E Incisura angularis.

Anatomically, the stomach can be divided into four regions. The cardia is the region where the oesophagus inserts into the stomach and food content is received. The fundus is the uppermost part and forms the upper curvature. The body is the main central region. The pylorus is the gastric outlet into the duodenum. The gastric antrum is the portion of the pylorus before the outlet. It does not produce acid. The incisura angularis is a well-defined notch in the lesser curvature of the stomach and serves as a landmark for identifying the lower extent of the body of the stomach.

7.15 Longitudinal ultrasound of the liver

A Ligamentum venosum.
B Left lobe of the liver.
C Common bile duct.
D Portal vein.
E Vertebrae.

The ligamentum venosum is the remnant of the ductus venosus of the foetal circulation, and appears as a hyperechoic stripe on ultrasound. It is normally attached to the left branch of the portal vein within the porta hepatis. It lies within a fissure between the caudate lobe and the left lobe of the liver, and serves as a useful landmark for identifying the caudate lobe on ultrasound.

The common hepatic artery is a short branch of the coeliac artery and typical divides into the left and right hepatic, right gastric and gastroduodenal arteries. The inferior vena cava lies to the right of the aorta and is the primary venous return to the heart.

7.16 Axial CT of the shoulder

A Right deltoid muscle.
B Right pectoralis minor muscle.
C Right pectoralis major muscle.
D Right humerus.
E Right triceps muscle.

The deltoid is the outermost muscle of the shoulder and is innervated by the axillary nerve. It is an abductor of the arm in the scapula plane.

The pectoralis major lies anterior to the pectoralis minor and arises from the medial half of the clavicle, the sternum and the cartilage of the true ribs. The fibres converge to join as a tendon attaching to the lateral lip of the bicipital groove of the humerus. The pectoralis major is innervated by the medial and lateral pectoral nerves.

The pectoralis minor arises from the third to the fifth ribs and inserts into the coracoid process of the scapula. It is innervated by the medial pectoral nerve. The triceps muscle has three heads – medial, lateral and long heads. The long head arises from the infraglenoid surface of the scapula. The medial and lateral heads insert to the dorsal aspect of the humerus.

7.17 Axial CT of the left knee

A Left medial patella facet.
B Left medial femoral condyle.
C Left lateral patella facet.
D Left medial patellar retinaculum.
E Left intercondylar notch.

The patella is the largest sesamoid bone in the body. The posterior surface is divided into medial and lateral facets. The medial facet is usually the smaller of the two. On MRI it is worth inspecting the facet surfaces for evidence of bone oedema as this can be a good marker for recent patella dislocation.

There are a few ways to work out which knee is being imaged when the side is not marked on the film. The position of the long saphenous vein is very helpful; it is seen on the left side of this image. Another good clue is that the medial patella facet is generally shorter and more vertical than the lateral patella facet. As CT orientation is standardized, it is therefore possible to tell that this image is of a left knee.

7.18 AP and oblique X-rays of a paediatric hand

A Right trapezium.
B Right scaphoid.
C Right hamate.
D Right lunate.
E Right ulna styloid.

There are eight carpal bones. A useful mnemonic for remembering them is:

Sally Left The Party To Take Cathy Home.

(From radial to ulna side, proximal row to distal row: scaphoid, lunate, triquetral, pisiform, trapezium, trapezoid, capitate, hamate.)

Please see Questions 2.17, 4.16 and 9.9 for more images and explanation of the carpal bones. A table of carpal bone ossification ages can be found in the answer to Question 10.13.

7.19 Coronal T1 MRI of the left wrist

A Extensor carpi ulnaris tendon.
B Triangular fibrocartilage.
C Ulna.
D Trapezium.
E Flexor digitorum profundus tendons.

The triangular fibrocartilage complex (TFCC) refers to the ligamentous and cartilaginous structures that lie between the ulna and the carpal bones (lunate and triquetrum). It is the major ligamentous stabilizer of the distal radio-ulnar joint and the ulna carpus, and acts to provide smooth gliding articulation of the wrist joint. The predominant component of the triangular fibrocartilage complex is a triangular wedge-shaped fibrocartilagenous disc bridging the distal radioulnar joint. The triangular fibrocartilage is a biconcave disc separating the radiocarpal and distal radioulnar joint spaces. It is the only structure of the triangular fibrocartilage complex consistently visualized on MRI.

7.20 Axial T1 MRI of the thighs

A Right sartorius muscle.
B Right long saphenous vein.
C Left adductor longus muscle.
D Right gracilis muscle.
E Right vastus medialis muscle.

The adductor canal (also known as Hunter's canal) is a musculo-fascial tunnel in the middle third of the medial thigh that contains the femoral vessels and saphenous nerve (as well as the nerve to vastus medialis). It is approximately 15 cm long and runs from the apex of the femoral triangle to the adductor hiatus.

Boundaries of the adductor canal:

Anterolateral	Vastus medialis
Posteromedial	Adductor longus, adductor magnus
Anterior	Sartorius

For more information and images of thigh anatomy, please see Questions 3.19, 5.17 and 6.19.

Examination 8: Questions

Question 8.1

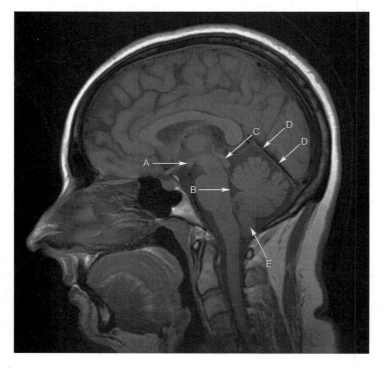

Name the structures labelled **A** to **E**.

Question 8.2

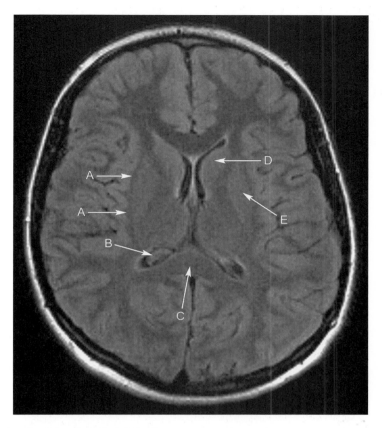

Name the structures labelled **A** to **E**.

Question 8.3

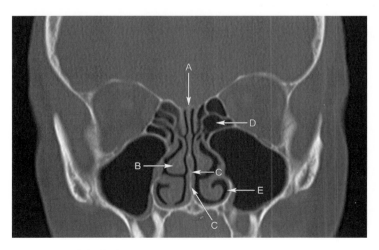

Name the structures labelled **A** to **E**.

Question 8.4

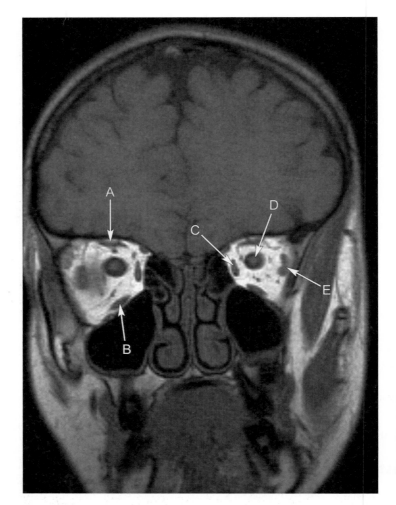

Name the structures labelled **A** to **E**.

Question 8.5

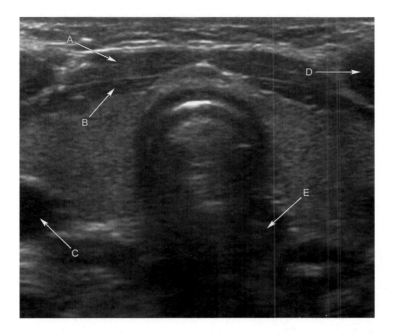

This is a transverse ultrasound of the neck.
Name the structures labelled **A** to **E**.

Question 8.6

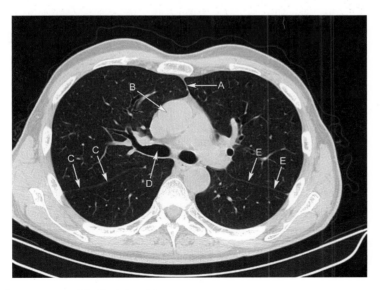

Name the structures labelled **A** to **E**.

Question 8.7

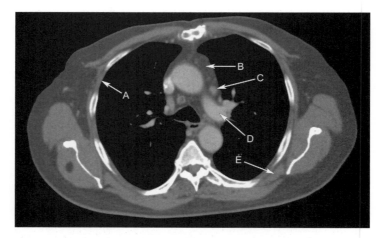

Name the structures labelled **A** to **E**.

Question 8.8

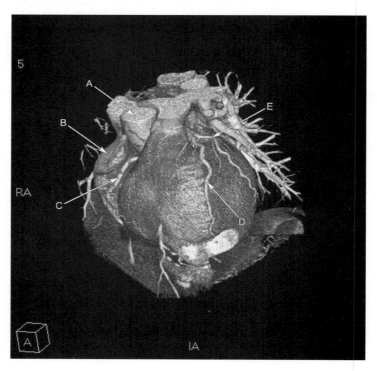

Name the structures labelled **A** to **E**.

Question 8.9

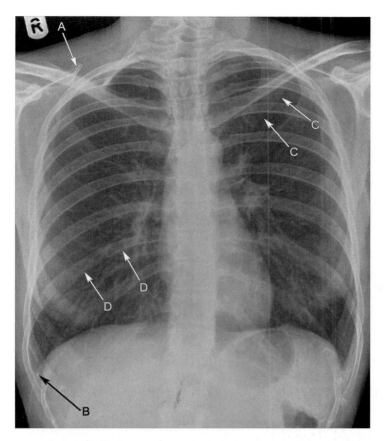

Name the structures labelled **A** to **D**.
E What normal variant is present?

Question 8.10

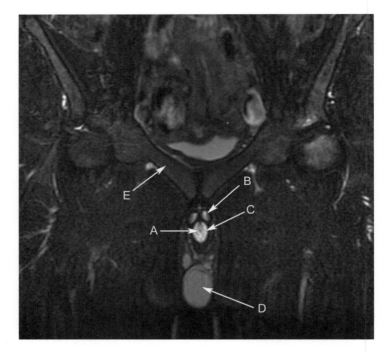

Name the structures labelled **A** to **E**.

Question 8.11

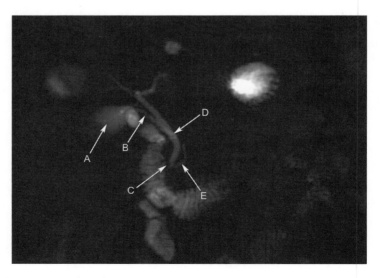

Name the structures labelled **A** to **E**.

Question 8.12

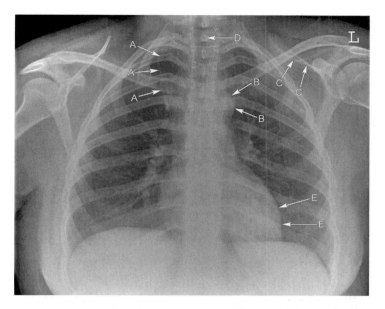

Name the structures labelled **A** to **E**.

Question 8.13

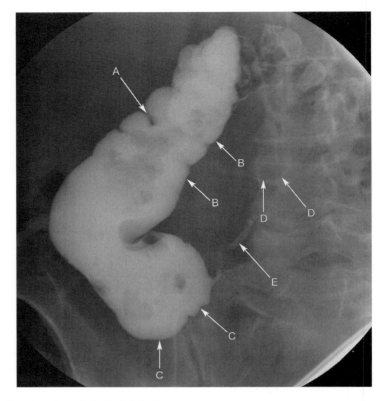

Name the structures labelled **A** to **E**.

Question 8.14

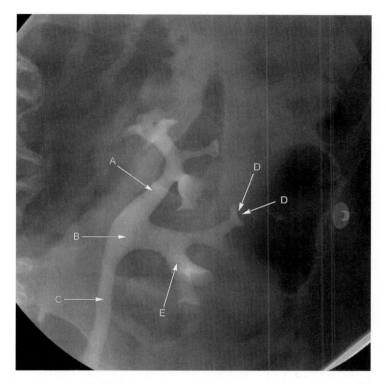

Name the structures labelled **A** to **E**.

Question 8.15

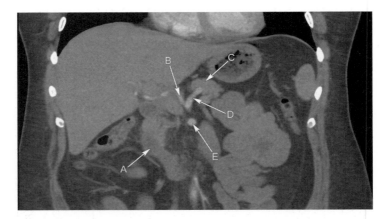

Name the structures labelled **A** to **E**.

Question 8.16

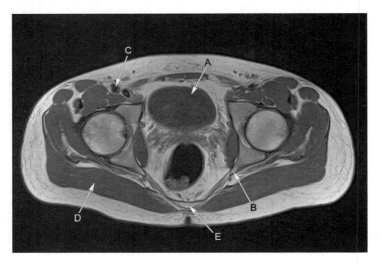

Name the structures labelled **A** to **E**.

Question 8.17

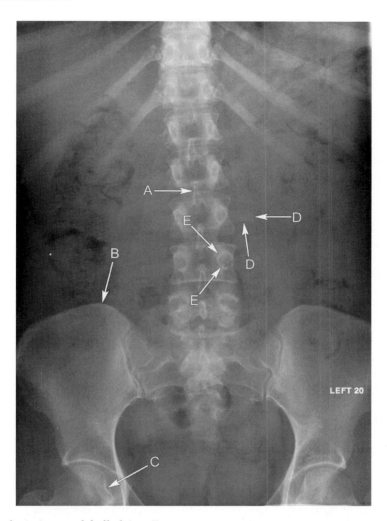

Name the structures labelled **A** to **E**.

Question 8.18

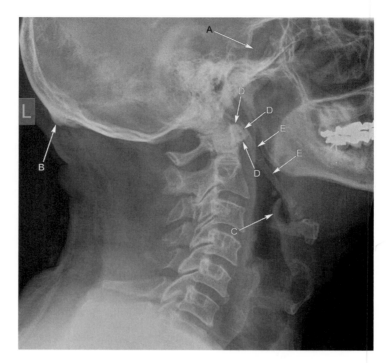

Name the structures labelled **A** to **D**.
E What normal variant is present?

Question 8.19

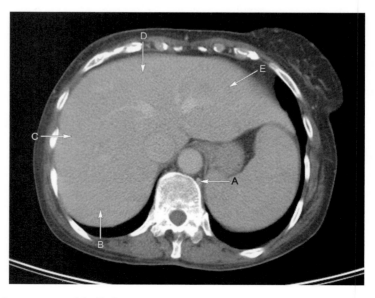

Name the structures labelled **A** to **E**.

Question 8.20

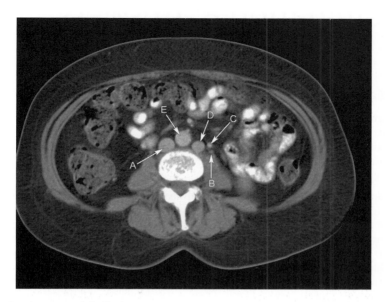

Name the structures labelled **A** to **E**.

Examination 8: Answers

8.1 Sagittal T1 MRI of the brain

A Mammillary body.
B Fourth ventricle.
C Tectum of the midbrain.
D Tentorium cerebelli.
E Cerebellar tonsil.

The mammillary bodies are a pair of rounded prominences at the anterior arches of the fornix. They are part of the limbic system. They can be damaged as a result of thiamine deficiency (Wernicke–Korsakoff syndrome). The fourth ventricle is the most inferior of the ventricular spaces and is diamond-shaped in cross section. It connects to the third ventricle via the aqueduct of Sylvius, and drains via the foramen of Luschka (two lateral tracts) and the foramen of Magendie (single midline tract). The tectum is located at the dorsal region of the midbrain and consists of superior (visual) and inferior (auditory) colliculi. There is a cerebellar tonsil on the undersurface of each cerebellar hemisphere in continuity with the uvula of the cerebellar vermis. It is helpful to assess these on sagittal section to look for elongation and descent of the cerebellar tonsils into the foramen magnum, which can be associated with raised intracranial pressure or congenital malformations (Chiari malformations).

8.2 Axial T2 FLAIR MRI of the brain

A Right external capsule.
B Choroid plexus in the right lateral ventricle.
C Splenium of the corpus callosum.
D Left caudate nucleus (head).
E Left lentiform nucleus.

The external capsule is a collection of white matter tracts seen lateral to the lentiform nucleus of each hemisphere. The lentiform nucleus (named after its shape) consists of two parts – globus pallidus (medial) and putamen (lateral). The caudate nucleus is C-shaped and consists of a head, body and tail. The head of the caudate nucleus forms part of the floor and wall of the anterior horn of the lateral ventricle. The caudate nucleus is separated from the lentiform nucleus by the anterior limb of the internal capsule.

8.3 Coronal CT of the sinuses

A Cribriform plate.
B Right middle turbinate.
C Nasal septum.
D Left ethmoid sinus.
E Left inferior meatus.

The nasal cavity is divided into two halves by the nasal septum. The nasal septum is formed by the perpendicular plate of the ethmoid bone, the septal cartilage and the vomer. The lateral walls of the nasal cavity are irregular due to the three turbinates (or conchae) – superior, middle and inferior. These divide the cavity into superior, middle and inferior meati, each lying underneath the turbinate of the corresponding name. Above the superior turbinate is the sphenoethmoidal recess.

Drainage connections into the nasal cavity:

Sphenoethmoid recess	Sphenoid air cells
Superior meatus	Posterior group of ethmoid air cells
Middle meatus	Anterior group of ethmoid air cells, frontal sinus
Inferior meatus	Nasolacrimal duct

The cribriform plate is part of the ethmoid bone and forms the central portion of the roof of the nasal cavity.

8.4 Coronal T1 MRI of the brain

A Right superior rectus muscle.
B Right inferior rectus muscle.
C Left medial rectus muscle.
D Left optic nerve.
E Left lateral rectus muscle.

There are six extrinsic ocular muscles controlling eye movement – four rectus muscles (superior, inferior, medial and lateral) and the superior and inferior oblique muscles. The rectus muscles share a common tendinous ring called the annulus of Zinn, and insert into the sclera of the orbit. The superior oblique muscle arises from the sphenoid bone superomedial to the optic foramen. The inferior oblique muscle arises from the anterior part of the orbital floor.

The following formula can help as a mnemonic to remember the innervation of the orbital nerves:

LR6SO4R3.

Lateral rectus	Sixth cranial nerve (abducens)
Superior oblique	Fourth cranial nerve (trochlear)
Rest of the muscles	Third cranial nerve (oculomotor)

8.5 Transverse ultrasound at the level of the thyroid isthmus

A Right sternohyoid muscle.
B Right sternothyroid muscle.
C Right common carotid artery.
D Left sternocleidomastoid muscle.
E Oesophagus.

The sternohyoid and sternothyroid are two of the four pairs of infrahyoid (strap) muscles. They are innervated by the ansa cervicalis (C1–C3). They serve to depress the hyoid bone. The sternocleidomastoid muscle anatomically divides the anterior and posterior triangles of the neck.

8.6 Axial high resolution CT (HRCT) of the chest

A Anterior junctional line.
B Ascending aorta.
C Right oblique fissure.

D Right main bronchus.
E Left oblique fissure.

The anterior junctional line is formed by the apposition of the visceral and parietal pleura of the lungs. In the right lung, the oblique fissure divides the lower lobe from the middle lobe. In the left lung, the oblique fissure divides the lower lobe from the upper lobe.

8.7 Axial CT of the chest with IV contrast

A Right intercostal muscle.
B Mediastinal fat.
C Lymph node in aorto-pulmonary window.
D Left main pulmonary artery.
E Left rhomboid major muscle.

There are three principal layers of intercostal muscle – external, internal and inner-most intercostal muscles. The neurovascular bundle runs in between the internal and innermost intercostal muscles. The rhomboid major muscle connects the scapula with the vertebrae and acts to retract and downwardly rotate the scapula.

8.8 3D reconstruction of a cardiac CT

A Ascending aorta.
B Right atrial appendage.
C Right coronary artery.
D Left anterior descending artery.
E Left circumflex artery.

The right atrial appendage is a small conical muscular pouch joined to the right atrium. It lies at the root of the ascending aorta, and the right coronary artery emerges from under it.

For further information about the coronary arteries, see Questions 3.6 and 7.8.

8.9 PA X-ray of the chest

A Superior angle of right scapula.
B Right costophrenic angle.
C Left anterior first rib.
D Right posterior ninth rib.
E Right cervical rib.

A cervical rib is an additional rib arising from the seventh cervical vertebra and is found in approximately 1 in 500 people. It is generally unilateral. Cervical ribs can be problematic and lead to thoracic outlet syndrome from compression of the brachial plexus or subclavian artery. These structures become trapped between the cervical rib and the scalene muscles. Symptoms include arm weakness and paraesthesia.

8.10 T2 FLAIR coronal MRI of the pelvis

A Urethra.
B Left corpus cavernosum.
C Corpus spongiosum.
D Testis.
E Right superior pubic ramus.

By convention, the ventral surface of the penis is the surface that normally lies upon the scrotum. There are three cylinders of epithelium-lined erectile tissue within the penis – a ventral corpus spongiosum and two dorsal corpus cavernosa. The three corpora generally give a high T2 signal on MRI.

There is a fibrous capsule surrounding each of the corpora, known as the tunica albuginea. A second fibrous layer, called Buck's fascia, surrounds the corpora cavernosa and separates them from the corpus spongiosum. As these two layers are both formed of dense fibrous tissue, they appear as a low-signal band on both T1- and T2-weighted MRI, and as such cannot be distinguished from each other. There is a layer of connective tissue superficial to Buck's fascia that has a relatively high T2 signal. Enveloping this is a further fascial layer called the tunica dartos, which is again T1 and T2 hypointense. The tunica dartos is a continuation of Scarpa's fascia, and is responsible for the wrinkled appearance of the scrotum.

8.11 MR cholangiopancreatography

A Gallbladder.
B Cystic duct.
C Ampulla of Vater (hepatopancreatic ampulla).
D Common bile duct.
E Pancreatic duct.

The common bile duct and pancreatic duct typically unite at the ampulla of Vater. This is located at the major duodenal papilla, halfway along the second part of the duodenum. This is an important point as is marks the transition from foregut to midgut, and is the point where arterial supply changes from the coeliac trunk to the superior mesenteric artery.

In a minority of people there is an additional dorsal pancreatic duct (the duct of Santorini) which usually drains separately into a second smaller (minor) papilla, approximately 2 cm proximal to the main papilla. The ventral pancreatic duct (the duct of Wirsung) continues to drain via the major papilla. This variant is termed pancreas divisum and is a risk factor for pancreatitis.

8.12 PA X-ray of the chest

A Azygos fissure.
B Aortic knuckle or arch.
C Spine of the left scapula.
D Spinous process of T2.
E Left ventricle.

The azygos fissure is a normal variant seen in 1–2% of individuals. It is formed when the azygos vein fails to migrate over the apex of the lung during foetal development. The azygos vein instead courses through the lung, bringing a layer of parietal and visceral pleura with it. The azygos fissure therefore consists of four layers of pleura (two parietal layers and two visceral layers). These wrap around the vein and are said to give a 'tadpole' appearance on the plain chest radiograph.

8.13 Barium enema

A Haustrum.
B Ascending colon.
C Caecal pole.

D Right pedicle of L4.
E Appendix.

The tenia coli are longitudinal ribbons of smooth muscle on the exterior of the colon. They are shorter than the bowel and contract longitudinally, causing the colon to become sacculated, forming the pouches known as haustra.

The position of the appendix is variable. Approximately 60% are retrocaecal and 35% are inferomedial.

8.14 Retrograde pyelogram of the left kidney

A Left upper pole infundibulum.
B Left renal pelvis.
C Left proximal ureter.
D Left lower pole fornix.
E Left lower pole major calyx.

A kidney generally comprises seven or eight pairs of minor calyces. The minor calyces combine to form two or three major calyces, which in turn drain via their infundibula to the renal pelvis.

For more information about the pelvicalyceal system see Question 5.15.

8.15 Coronal CT of the abdomen with IV contrast

A Second part of the duodenum.
B Common hepatic artery.
C Pancreas.
D Splenic artery.
E Superior mesenteric artery.

The duodenum forms a C shape around the head of the pancreas and is divided anatomically into four parts. The first part (duodenal cap) passes superiorly, to the right and posterior of the pylorus. It may be indented by the gallbladder. The second part is roughly vertical and is the site of insertion of the ampulla of Vater. The third part curves anteriorly around the inferior vena cava, aorta and L3 vertebra. The head of the pancreas is in contact with its superior border. It is indented by the aorta posteriorly and the superior mesenteric artery and vein superiorly. The fourth part of the duodenum continues to pass to the left of midline to reach the duodenal-jejunal junction. The ligament of Treitz lies at the highest part of the fourth part of duodenum.

The common hepatic artery and splenic artery both arise from the coeliac trunk. The superior mesenteric artery lies to the left of the superior mesenteric vein.

See Question 1.14 for further descriptions of the duodenal anatomy.

8.16 Axial T1 MRI of the pelvis

A Bladder.
B Left ischial spine.
C Right femoral artery.
D Right gluteus maximus.
E Sacrum.

The ischial spine is a triangular eminence from the posterior border of the ischium. It gives rise to the superior gemellus muscle on its external surface and the coccygeus, levator ani and pelvic fascia on its internal surface. The sacrospinous ligament attaches to its pointed apex. The pudendal nerve passes dorsal to the ischial spine. For this reason the ischial spine can serve as a useful landmark for performing a pudendal nerve block.

8.17 AP X-ray of the abdomen

A Spinous process of L2.
B Right posterior superior iliac spine/right ilium.
C Right fovea capitis.
D Left transverse process of L3.
E Left pedicle of L4.

The fovea capitis is a depression on the anterosuperior part of head of femur giving rise to the ligamentum teres.

The two pedicles and the spinous process resemble the appearance of an owl. The 'winking owl' sign refers to the erosion of a pedicle by a lytic process, such as metastatic disease.

8.18 Lateral X-ray of the cervical spine

A Sphenoid sinus.
B External occipital protuberance.
C Epiglottis.
D Anterior arch of C1.
E Calcified stylohyoid ligament.

The stylohyoid ligament is at the superior end of the stylohyoid muscle and connects to the styloid process of the temporal bone. It is not uncommon for this ligament to be partially ossified, as is seen on this image. This can lead to the formation of an elongated styloid process, which is seen in approximately 4% of the population. In a small percentage of these people (5–10%) this elongation is believed to be the cause of a cluster of symptoms including throat pain, globus, dysphagia, tinnitus and facial pain. This is known as Eagle's syndrome, described by Watt Weems Eagle in 1937. Stylohyoid calcification (with or without styloid process elongation) has also been described in the literature as a potential cause of difficult intubation, so if present it is well worth noting the finding in the report.

8.19 Axial CT of the abdomen with IV contrast

A Hemiazygos vein.
B Segment VII of the liver.
C Segment VIII of the liver.
D Segment IVa of the liver.
E Segment II of the liver.

In 1957, Couinaud described the liver as containing eight discrete functionally independent segments. Each segment has its own vascular inflow (branch of the portal vein), outflow (branch of the hepatic vein) and biliary drainage. The portal vein divides the liver into upper and lower segments. The caudate lobe is segment I. Segment IV is often subdivided into IVa (superior) and IVb (inferior).

For a diagram of the liver segments, please see Question 10.5.

8.20 Axial CT of the abdomen with IV and oral contrast

A Right inferior vena cava.
B Left ureter.
C Left gonadal vein.
D Left inferior vena cava.
E Aorta.

This patient has a double inferior vena cava, which is an uncommon abnormality with a prevalence of 0.2–3%. It results from persistence of both supracardinal veins during embryogenesis (normally the left supracardinal vein regresses or fuses with the right supracardinal vein). A double inferior vena cava should be suspected in cases of recurrent pulmonary embolism despite the deployment of a caval filter.

Examination 9: Questions

Question 9.1

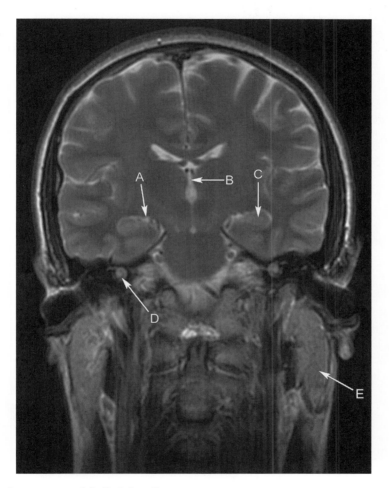

Name the structures labelled **A** to **E**.

Question 9.2

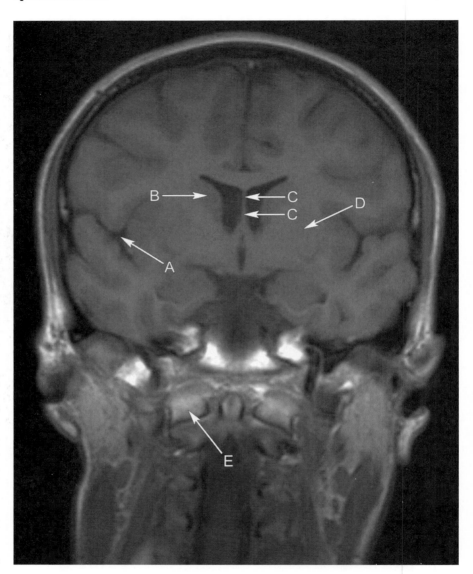

Name the structures labelled **A** to **E**.

Question 9.3

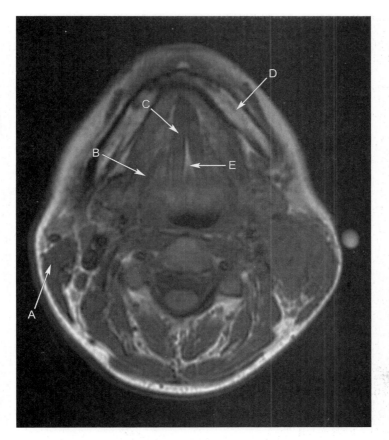

Name the structures labelled **A** to **E**.

Question 9.4

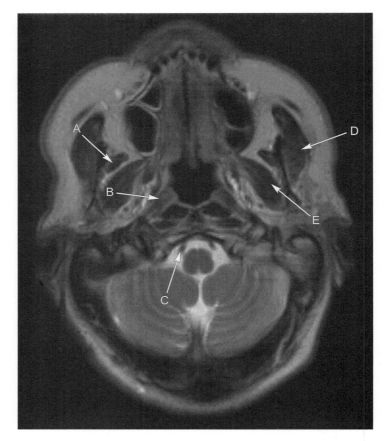

Name the structures labelled **A** to **E**.

Question 9.5

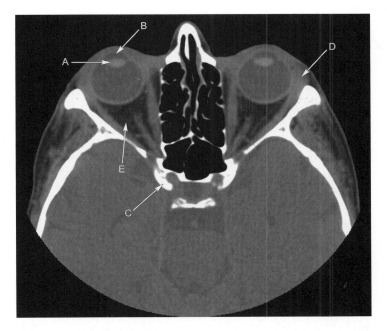

Name the structures labelled **A** to **E**.

Question 9.6

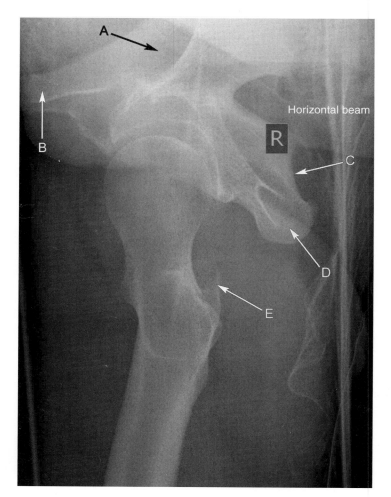

Name the structures labelled **A** to **E**.

Question 9.7

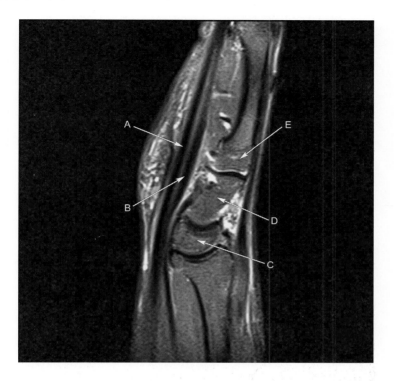

This is an MRI of the right wrist.
Name the structures labelled **A** to **E**.

Question 9.8

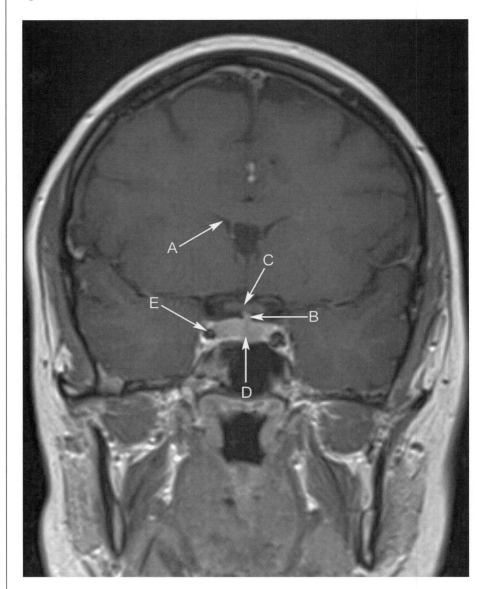

Name the structures labelled **A** to **E**.

Question 9.9

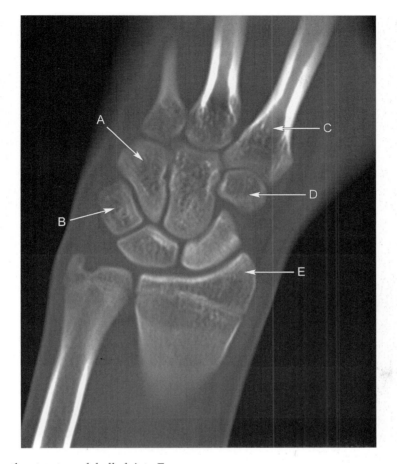

Name the structures labelled **A** to **E**.

Question 9.10

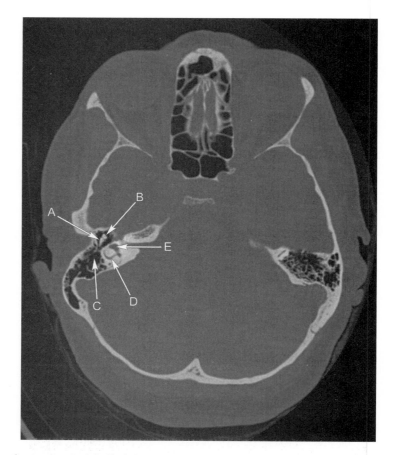

Name the structures labelled **A** to **E**.

Question 9.11

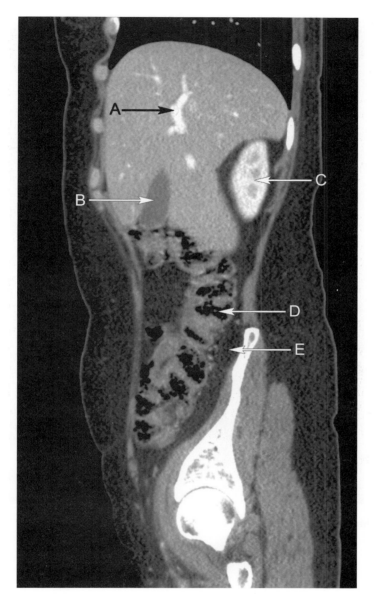

Name the structures labelled **A** to **E**.

Question 9.12

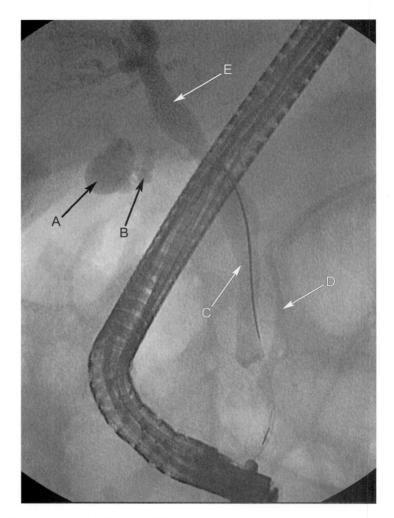

Name the structures labelled **A** to **E**.

Question 9.13

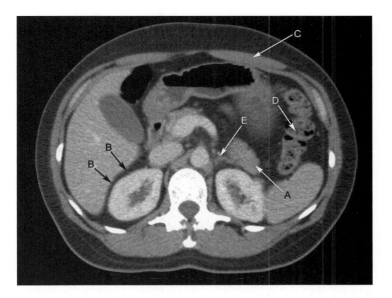

Name the structures labelled **A** to **E**.

Question 9.14

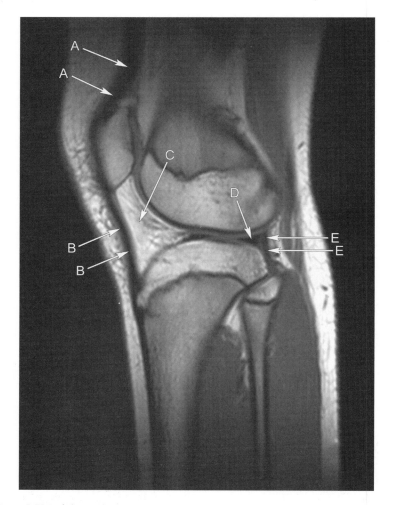

This is an MRI of the right knee.
Name the structures labelled **A** to **E**.

Question 9.15

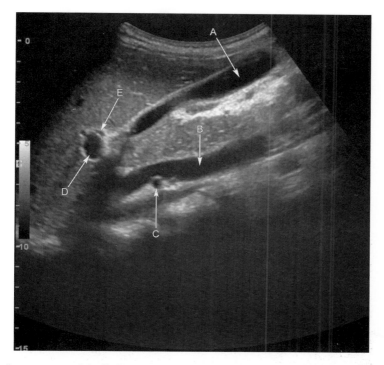

Name the structures labelled **A** to **E**.

Question 9.16

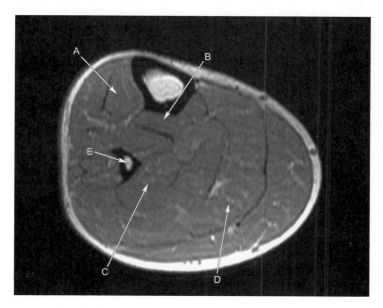

This is an axial MRI of the lower leg.
Name the structures labelled **A** to **E**.

Question 9.17

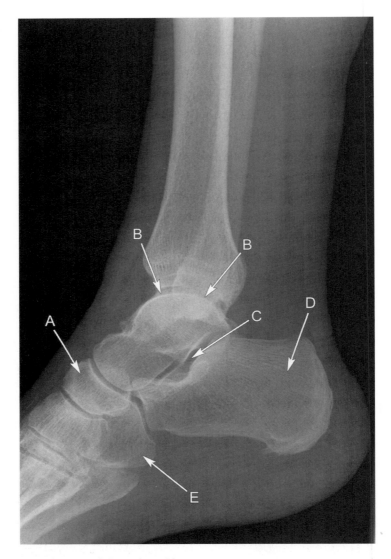

This is a lateral X-ray of the right ankle.
Name the structures labelled **A** to **E**.

Question 9.18

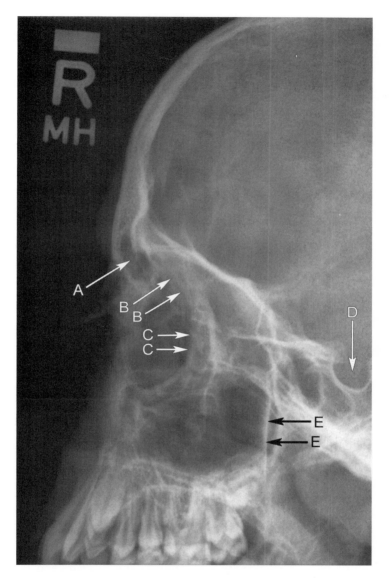

Name the structures labelled **A** to **E**.

Question 9.19

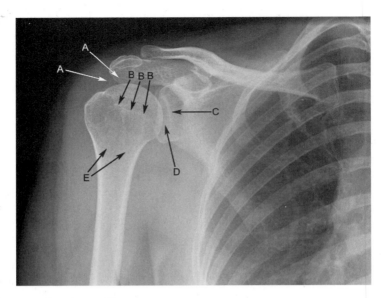

A What muscle is located here?
Name the structures labelled **B** to **E**.

Question 9.20

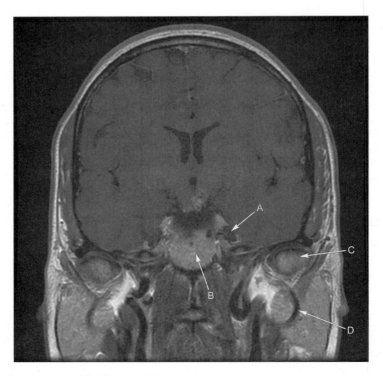

Name the structures labelled **A** to **D**.
E What structure is located in A?

Examination 9: Answers

9.1 Coronal T2 MRI of the brain

A Temporal horn of right lateral ventricle.
B Third ventricle.
C Left hippocampus.
D Right cochlea.
E Left parotid gland.

The lateral ventricles drain cerebrospinal fluid into the third ventricle via the right and left interventricular foramen (foramen of Munro). The third ventricle drains into the fourth ventricle via the cerebral aqueduct (aqueduct of Sylvius). The fourth ventricle drains via a central foramen of Magendie and two lateral foramina of Luschka.

The hippocampus is a key part of the limbic system and is seen as a curved prominence on the inferior horn of the lateral ventricle. It is a grey-matter structure with a thin covering of white matter, which is known as the alveus.

For more information and a flow diagram of the ventricular system see Question 4.2.

9.2 Coronal T1 MRI of the brain

A Right sylvian fissure.
B Right caudate nucleus.
C Septum pellucidum.
D Left putamen.
E Right lateral mass of C1.

The septum pellucidum is a thin membrane separating the anterior horns of the lateral ventricles. It consists of two layers of both white and grey matter, called the laminae septi pellucidi. During foetal development there is a space between these two laminae called the cavum septum pellucidum. This is fused in 85% of individuals by six months of age but can persist into adulthood as a normal variant.

For an example of a cavum septum pellucidum see Question 9.8.

9.3 Axial T1 MRI of the neck

A Right sternocleidomastoid muscle.
B Right hyoglossus muscle.
C Right genioglossus muscle.
D Body of left mandible.
E Lingual septum.

The hyoglossus muscle runs from the hyoid bone vertically upwards to the side of the tongue (between the styloglossus and the longitudinalis inferior). It acts to depress and retract the tongue.

The genioglossus muscle passes from the mental spine of the mandible to the hyoid bone and dorsum of the tongue. It acts to depress and protrude the tongue.

Both of these muscles are innervated by the hypoglossal nerve (CN XII).

9.4 Axial T1 MRI of the neck

A Right temporalis muscle.
B Right levator veli palatini muscle.
C Right vertebral artery.
D Left masseter.
E Left lateral pterygoid muscle.

The temporalis, medial pterygoid, lateral pterygoid and masseter muscles are the four muscles of mastication. They are all innervated by the mandibular branch of the trigeminal nerve (CN V^3). The temporalis muscle runs from the temporal fossa to the coronoid process of the mandible. The lateral pterygoid runs from the infratemporal surface of the sphenoid bone (upper head) and the lateral surface of the lateral pterygoid plate (lower head) to the pterygoid fovea below the mandibular condyle. The masseter muscle runs from the zygomatic arch to the angle of the mandible.

The levator veli palatine muscle acts to elevate and retract the soft palate and is supplied primarily by the vagus nerve (CN X).

9.5 Axial CT of the orbits

A Right lens.
B Right cornea.
C Right anterior clinoid process.
D Inferior pole of the left lacrimal gland.
E Right intraconal fat.

The cornea is the transparent structure at the front of the eye overlying the iris, pupil and lens. It has no blood supply. The aqueous humour is a thick watery substance containing amino acids that lies in between the cornea and the lens. A disruption of its normal circulation can lead to glaucoma.

The orbital septum is a membranous fascia, which acts as the anterior boundary to the orbit. It lies between the orbital rim and the tarsus, making up the fibrous component of the eyelids.

The lacrimal gland is a bilobed gland lying in the superotemporal orbit within the lacrimal fossa.

9.6 Lateral X-ray of the hip

A Right obturator foramen.
B Right superior pubic ramus.
C Right lesser sciatic notch.
D Right ischial tuberosity.
E Right greater trochanter.

The obturator foramen is formed by the ischium and pubis bones. The obturator canal passes through this and contains the obturator artery, nerve and vein. The lesser sciatic notch is covered by the sacrotuberous and sacrospinous ligaments to become the lesser sciatic foramen. This foramen transmits the obturator internus tendon and nerve, and the internal pudendal vessels and nerve. The ischial tuberosity gives rise to the adductor magnus, the semimembranosis, the long head of the biceps femoris, the semitendinosis and the sacrotuberous ligament.

9.7 Sagittal STIR MRI of the right wrist

A Tendon of flexor digitorum superficialis.
B Tendon of flexor digitorum profundus.

C Lunate.
D Capitate.
E Base of the third metacarpal.

The tendons of the flexor digitorum profundus (FDP) run deep to the tendons of the flexor digitorum superficialis (FDS), and insert distally to the tendons of the flexor digitorum superficialis. The four tendons of the flexor digitorum superficialis (one for each finger apart from the thumb) each divide to allow passage of the tendons of the flexor digitorum profundus and then reunite distally to insert into the palmar aspect of the bases of the second to the fifth middle phalanges. The tendons of the flexor digitorum profundus continue to insert into the palmar aspect of the base of the second to the fifth distal phalanges.

For an explanation of the alignment of the carpal bones in the sagittal plane see Question 4.16.

9.8 Coronal T1 MRI of the brain with IV contrast

A Right lateral ventricle.
B Infundibulum (pituitary stalk).
C Optic chiasm.
D Pituitary gland.
E Right internal carotid artery.

The pituitary gland lies within the sella turcica, which is covered by a dural fold called the diaphragma sellae. It is connected to the hypothalamus by a thin process called the infundibulum (or pituitary stalk). The pituitary gland is generally divided into two sections – anterior (adenohypophysis) and posterior (neurohypophysis). There is a further intermediate section, but this is only a few cells thick and is generally included with the anterior pituitary.

At birth, the pituitary gland is globular in shape and exhibits a generalized high signal on T1-weighted MRI. By six weeks of age this high signal has largely diminished in the anterior lobe, which returns an isointense signal similar to brain parenchyma. The posterior pituitary continues to display a high signal on T1-weighted MRI, giving rise to the characteristic posterior pituitary bright spot. This normal finding is said to be related to the high neurophysin content of the posterior pituitary. The adult pituitary gland is normally 3–8 mm in height, and is generally larger in females.

Anatomical relations to the pituitary gland:

Superior	Optic chiasm (within suprasellar cistern)
Lateral	Cavernous sinuses (walls of the pituitary fossa)
Anteroposterior	Sphenoid sinus

This image displays an incidental finding of a cavum septum pellucidum.

9.9 Coronal CT of the wrist

A Right hamate.
B Right triquetral.
C Right second metacarpal.
D Right trapezoid.
E Right radial styloid.

For a table of the carpal bone ossification ages, please see Question 10.13.

9.10 Axial CT of the auditory canal

A Right incus.
B Right malleus.
C Right mastoid air cells.
D Right semicircular canal.
E Right vestibule.

The middle ear is a cavity in the petrous bone between the tympanic membrane and the inner ear. The upper part of the cavity is known as the attic and it communicates with the mastoid air cells through a posterior opening known as the aditus ad antrum. Three bony ossicles traverse the middle ear cavity – the malleus, incus and stapes. They are connected via synovial joints. On axial CT the appearance of the incus and malleus is sometimes described as an 'ice cream cone', with the malleus being the 'ice-cream' on top of the incus' 'cone'.

The bony labyrinth lies within the inner ear and consists of the vestibule, cochlear and three semicircular canals.

9.11 Sagittal CT of the abdomen with IV contrast

A Portal vein.
B Gallbladder.
C Right kidney.
D Ascending colon.
E Retroperitoneal fat.

The kidneys are retroperitoneal structures lying approximately at the level of T12 to L3. The right kidney is slightly lower than the left. The right kidney sits posterior to the liver just below the diaphragm. The upper parts of the kidneys lie partially under the eleventh and twelfth ribs. The kidneys are surrounded by two layers of fat (perirenal and pararenal fat) and Gerota's fascia.

9.12 ERCP

A Gallbladder.
B Cystic duct.
C Common bile duct.
D Pancreatic duct.
E Common hepatic duct.

The cystic duct is normally 2–4 cm long with a variable diameter from 1 to 5 mm. Its insertion into the extrahepatic bile duct marks the change from the common hepatic duct to the common bile duct. This point is usually halfway between the porta-hepatis and the ampulla of Vater.

The normal pancreatic diameter is up to 3 mm at the head of the pancreas, and around 2 mm distally.

9.13 Axial CT of the abdomen with IV contrast

A Tail of the pancreas.
B Hepatorenal recess (Morison's pouch).
C Left rectus abdominis muscle.
D Transverse colon.
E Left adrenal gland.

Morison's pouch is the eponymous name for the hepatorenal recess, a potential space separating the liver from the right kidney. It was described by a British surgeon named James Rutherford Morison (1853–1939). The hepatorenal recess is clinically important as fluid can collect here in the presence of ascites and haemoperitoneum. For this reason it is routinely assessed during FAST scanning of trauma patients.

9.14 Sagittal T1 MRI of the right knee

A Quadriceps tendon.
B Patella tendon.
C Hoffa's fat pad (infrapatella fat pad).
D Posterior horn of the lateral meniscus.
E Tendon of popliteus.

The quadriceps tendon inserts into the superior patella and is formed by the convergence of the four quadriceps muscles (the vastus intermedius, vastus medialis, vastus lateralis and rectus femoris).

The patella tendon runs from the apex and the posterior surface of the patella to the tibial tuberosity. The posterior surface of the patella tendon is separated from the synovial membrane of the joint by the infrapatella fat pad (known as Hoffa's fat pad).

The medial and lateral menisci of the knee are cartilaginous structures, which act to deepen the articular surface of the tibial plateau and contribute to the structural integrity of the knee during flexion and extension. The medial and lateral menisci are anatomically and functionally different from each other. Some key differences are outlined below:

1. The medial meniscus is C-shaped, and the lateral is closer to circular (O-shaped).
2. The posterior horn of the medial meniscus is much wider than the anterior horn. The lateral meniscus has almost uniform width.
3. The medial meniscus attaches to the joint capsule and deep fibres of the medial collateral ligament. The lateral meniscus attaches to the joint capsule but does not attach to the lateral collateral ligament. It does, however, have an additional attachment to the medial femoral condyle via meniscofemoral ligaments.
4. The lateral meniscus is normally twice as mobile as the medial meniscus (up to 10 mm movement physiologically).

Both menisci normally give a low signal on both T1- and T2-weighted MRI. It is more common to injure the medial meniscus than the lateral meniscus.

9.15 Longitudinal ultrasound of the abdomen

A Gallbladder.
B Inferior vena cava.
C Right renal artery.
D Portal vein.
E Common hepatic duct.

Since the aorta lies to the left of the inferior vena cava, the right renal artery is usually longer than the left. The right renal artery arises from the aorta at vertebral level L1 and passes behind the inferior cava, right renal vein, the head of the pancreas and the descending part of the duodenum before reaching the right kidney. There are several normal variants in renal artery anatomy. The most common of these is multiple renal arteries supplying one kidney, which occurs in 25–40% of the population.

9.16 T1 MRI of the lower leg

A Right tibialis anterior muscle.
B Right tibialis posterior muscle.
C Right flexor hallucis longus muscle.
D Right soleus muscle.
E Right fibula.

The lower leg is divided into four fascial compartments with separate nerve and blood supplies:

Superficial posterior (medial sural nerve)	Gastrocnemius; soleus; plantaris
Deep posterior (tibial nerve)	Tibialis posterior; flexor hallucis longus; flexor digitorum longus; popliteus
Anterior (deep peroneal nerve)	Tibialis anterior; extensor hallucis longus; extensor digitorum longus; peroneus tertius
Lateral (superficial peroneal nerve)	Peroneus brevis; peroneus longus

9.17 Lateral X-ray of the right ankle

A Navicular.
B Talar dome.
C Subtalar joint.
D Calcaneous.
E Cuboid.

There are seven tarsal bones in each foot: the talus, calcaneus, navicular, cuboid and three cuneiform bones. The talus and calcaneus form the hindfoot and the cuboid, navicular and cuneiforms form the midfoot.

The subtalar joint is the articulation between the talus and the calcaneus and allows inversion and eversion of the foot.

For further descriptions of the bony anatomy of the feet see Question 1.20.

9.18 Lateral X-ray of the facial bones

A Frontal sinus.
B Zygomatic process of the frontal bone.
C Frontal process of the zygomatic bone.
D Pituitary fossa.
E Posterior wall of the maxillary sinus.

The frontozygomatic suture lies in the region of the superolateral orbital margin. It is the point where the zygomatic process of the frontal bone meets the frontal process of the zygomatic bone.

9.19 AP X-ray of the shoulder

A Right supraspinatous muscle/tendon/subacromial joint space.
B Anatomical neck of the right humerus.
C Right glenoid.
D Right glenohumeral joint.
E Right surgical neck of the humerus.

The anatomical neck of the humerus is an oblique indentation distal to the humeral head where the joint articular capsule attaches. The upper outer part of it is seen as a groove separating the head from the greater tubercle of the humerus. The surgical neck of the humerus is a narrowing of the shaft below the lesser and greater tubercle – fractures are far more common here than the anatomical neck of the humerus.

The glenohumeral joint is a multiaxial synovial ball and socket joint. The glenoid fossa itself is shallow and is reinforced by the glenoid labrum to deepen it and increase joint stability.

The supraspinatous muscle is part of the rotator cuff and acts to abduct the shoulder joint. It originates in the supraspinous fossa and its tendon passes under the acromion through the supraspinatous outlet, finally inserting onto the greater tuberosity of the humerus. The supraspinatous outlet is formed by the acromion, coracoacromial arch, acromioclavicular joint, glenoid and humeral head. Abnormality of the outlet can lead to supraspinatous impingement and rotator cuff tendonitis. The supraspinatous tendon can be examined with both ultrasound and MRI. There are also dedicated X-ray views for assessing the supraspinatous outlet:

Stryker notch view	Looks for os acromiale
Supraspinatous outlet view	Useful for measuring subacromial space (<7mm = increased risk of impingement) Good for assessing morphology of acromion

9.20 Coronal FLAIR MRI of the brain

A Left Meckel's cave.
B Clivus.
C Left mandibular condyle.
D Terminal branch of the left external carotid artery.
E Left trigeminal ganglion.

Meckel's cave is a cerebrospinal fluid filled space lying immediately lateral to the cavernous sinus. It is bounded by dura overlying four structures:

Superolateral	Cerebellar tentorium
Superomedial	Lateral wall of the cavernous sinus
Medial	Clivus
Inferolateral	Posterior petrous

The trigeminal nerve (CN V) enters it through a defect in the dura and then expands to form the trigeminal (Gasserian) ganglion, which gives rise to the three branches of the trigeminal nerve.

Examination 10: Questions

Question 10.1

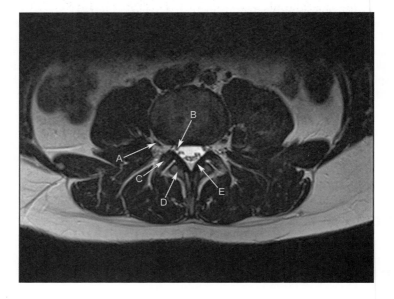

This is an MRI of the lumbar spine at the level of the L4/5 intervertebral disc. Name the structures labelled **A** to **E**.

Question 10.2

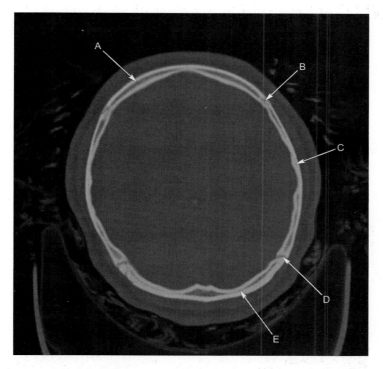

Name the structures labelled **A** to **E**.

Question 10.3

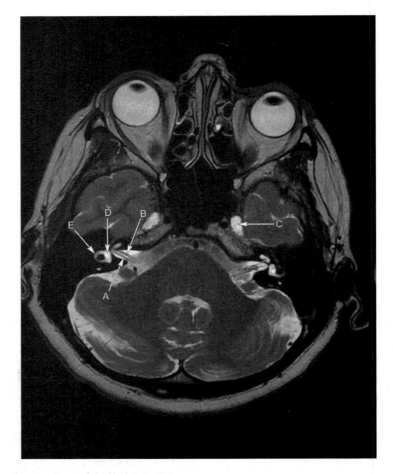

Name the structures labelled **A** to **E**.

Question 10.4

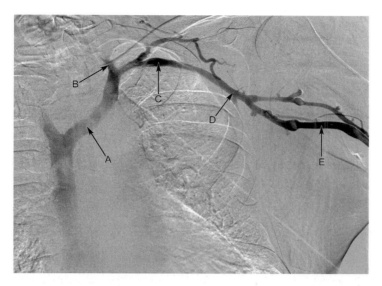

Name the structures labelled **A** to **E**.

Question 10.5

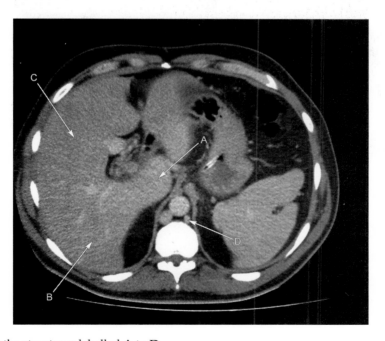

Name the structures labelled **A** to **D**.
E What normal variant is present?

Question 10.6

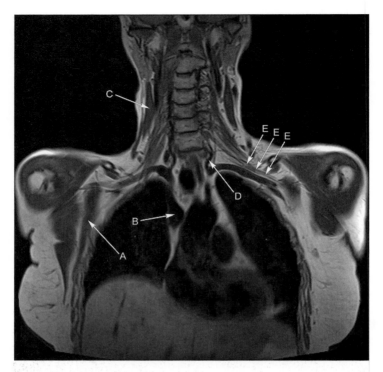

Name the structures labelled **A** to **E**.

Question 10.7

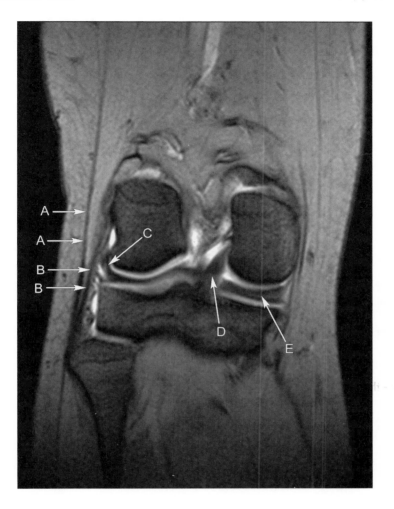

This is a coronal MRI of the right knee.
Name the structures labelled **A** to **E**.

Question 10.8

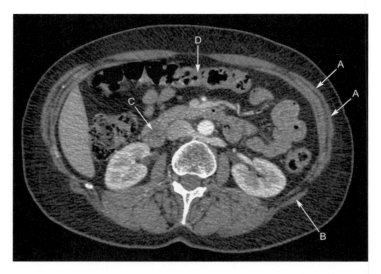

Name the structures labelled **A** to **D**.
E What normal variant is present?

Question 10.9

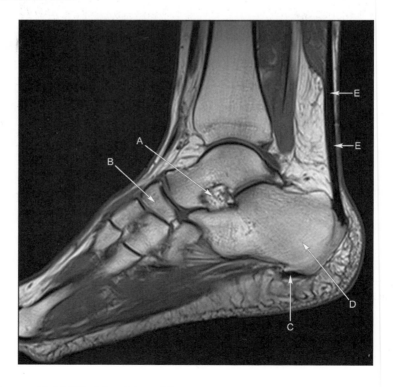

This is a sagittal MRI of the right ankle.
Name the structures labelled **A** to **E**.

Question 10.10

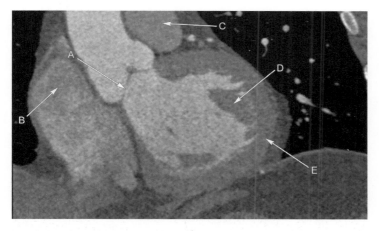

Name the structures labelled **A** to **E**.

Question 10.11

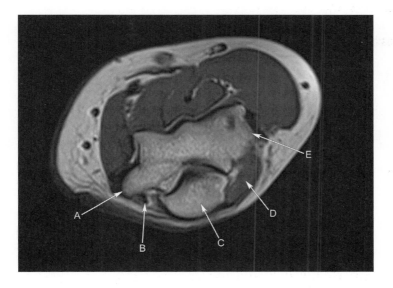

This is an axial MRI of the left elbow.
A Which shared tendon inserts here?
Name the structures labelled **B** to **D**.
E Which shared tendon inserts here?

Question 10.12

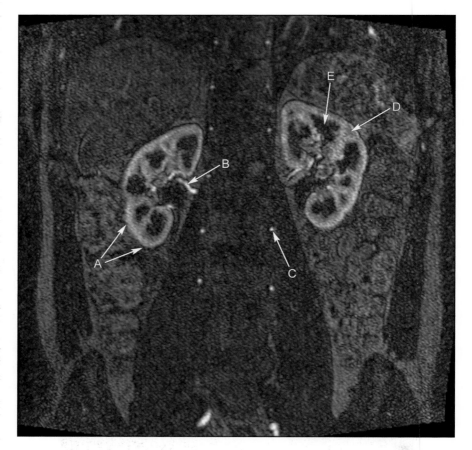

Name the structures labelled **A** to **E**.

Question 10.13

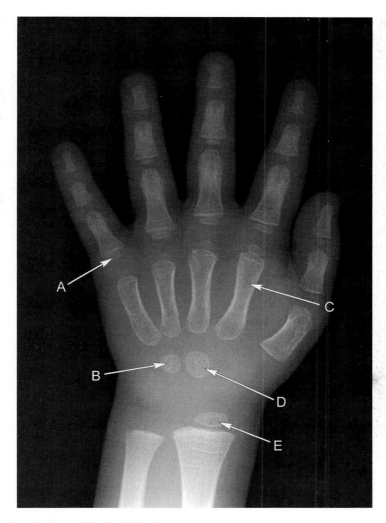

Name the structures labelled **A** to **E**.

Question 10.14

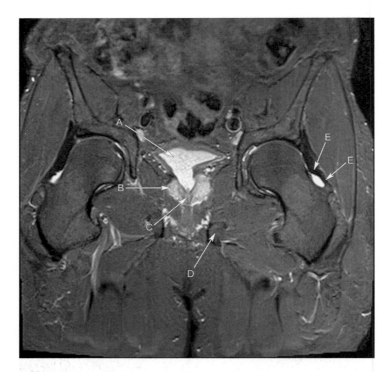

Name the structures labelled **A** to **E**.

Question 10.15

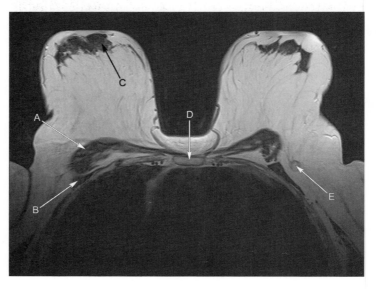

Name the structures labelled **A** to **E**.

Question 10.16

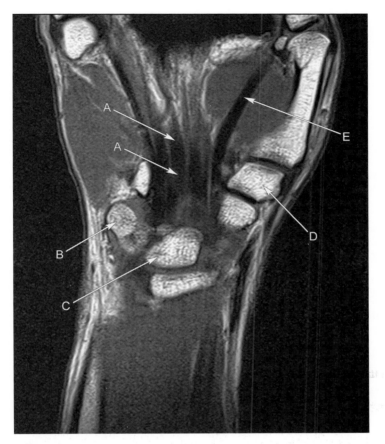

This is a coronal MRI of the right wrist.
Name the structures labelled **A** to **E**.

Question 10.17

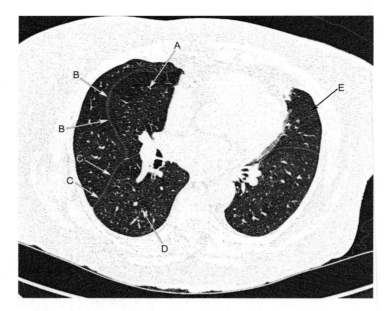

Name the structures labelled **A** to **E**.

Question 10.18

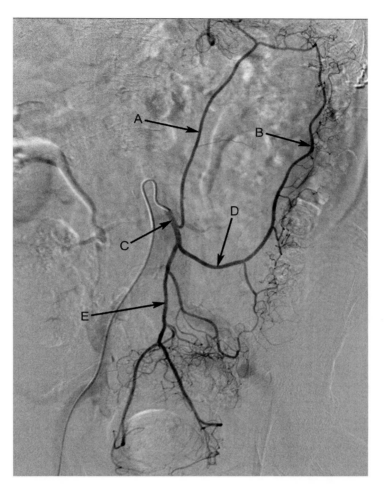

Name the structures labelled **A** to **E**.

Question 10.19

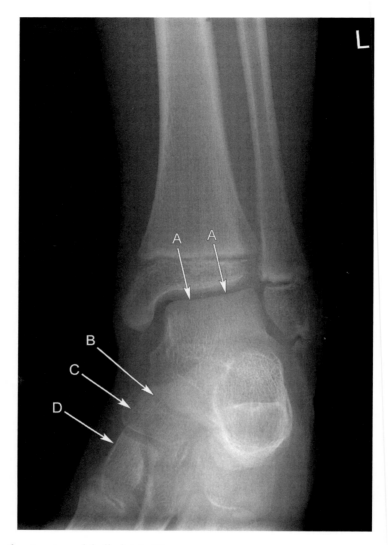

Name the structures labelled **A** to **D**.
E What normal variant is present?

Question 10.20

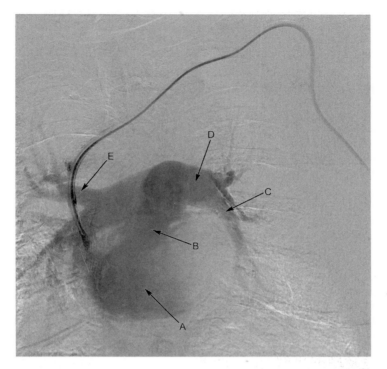

Name the structures labelled **A** to **E**.

Examination 10: Answers

10.1 Axial T2 MRI of the lumbar spine

A Right L4 exiting nerve root.
B Right L5 nerve root.
C Right superior articular facet of L5.
D Right inferior articular facet of L4.
E Ligamentum flavum.

The nerves of the cauda equina are well demonstrated on T2-weighted axial imaging of the lumbar spine. They appear as low signal intensity punctate structures within the bright signal intensity of the surrounding cerebrospinal fluid. The cauda equina are the continuing nerve roots from the cord, which gradually decrease in number as the root pairs exit the spinal column. Within the thoracolumbar spine the nerve roots exit at the exit foramen below the root. For example, the L4 nerve root exits at L4/L5, and is the traversing nerve root at L3/L4.

The ligamentum flavum is a collection of ligaments attached to the vertebral laminae running all the way from C2 to S1. They are seen posteriorly on the interior of the vertebral canal. Hypertrophy of these ligaments can lead to canal stenosis. The facet joints are well demonstrated on this image, with the inferior facets of the vertebra above (L4) lying posterior to the superior facets of the vertebra below (L5).

10.2 Axial CT of the skull

A Frontal bone.
B Left coronal suture.
C Left parietal bone.
D Left lambdoid suture.
E Occipital bone.

The skull is composed of 22 bones, each of which is joined together by sutures (fibrous joints which permit a minute amount of movement). Eight of these bones make up the skull vault, which forms a protective covering for the brain. These are:

- Two parietal bones.
- Two temporal bones.
- One frontal bone.
- One occipital bone.
- One sphenoid bone.
- One ethmoid bone.

The frontal bone articulates with the paired parietal bones via the coronal suture and forms the forehead as well as the roof and the lateral walls of the orbits. The paired parietal bones articulate with each other via the sagittal suture, with the frontal bone via the coronal suture and with the occipital bone via the lambdoid suture.

10.3 Axial T2 MRI of the brain

A Vestibulocochlear nerve (CN VIII).
B Facial nerve (CN VII).

C Left Meckel's cave.
D Right vestibule.
E Right semicircular canal.

The internal auditory meatus (IAM) is a short channel through the petrous temporal bone, which provides a passage from the posterior cranial fossa to the auditory apparatus. The contents of the IAM include the vestibulocochlear nerve (CN VIII), facial nerve (CN VII) and the labyrinthine artery. Bill's bar is a vertical bony ridge, which divides the IAM into an anterior and posterior component. The falciform crescent (or transverse crest) is a horizontal ridge, which divides the IAM into superior and inferior components.

The vestibulocochlear nerve is divided into the cochlear nerve and the vestibular nerve. The vestibular nerve is further subdivided into superior and inferior branches. The facial nerve has a motor component and a sensory component (nervus intermedius). The following schematic shows the arrangement of the nerves within a cross-section of the IAM.

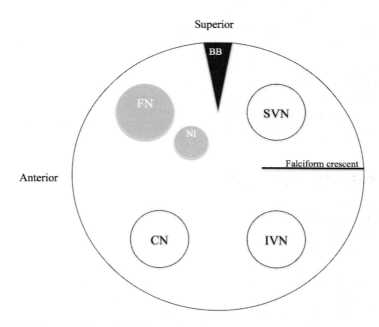

Figure 10.1 Cross-section of the internal auditory meatus: FN = facial nerve motor branch; NI = nervus intermedius (facial nerve sensory branch); CN = cochlear nerve; SVN = superior vestibular nerve (branch of vestibulocochlear nerve); IVN = inferior vestibular nerve (branch of vestibulocochlear nerve); BB = Bill's bar. A useful way to remember the positions of the nerves is '7-up, **C**oke Down', which refers to the facial nerve (**7th** nerve) and the **C**ochlear nerve.

10.4 Venogram of the left arm

A Left brachiocephalic (innominate) vein.
B Left internal jugular vein.
C Left subclavian vein.
D Left axillary vein.
E Left basilic vein.

The brachial veins are paired deep veins, which ascend on either side of the brachial artery in the upper arm. At the level of the teres major they join to form the axillary vein, which then continues to the lateral border of the first rib. At this point the name changes to the subclavian vein. The subclavian vein continues to the level of the clavicular head where it joins with the internal jugular vein to form the brachiocephalic vein, which in turn joins with the contralateral brachiocephalic vein to form the superior vena cava.

10.5 Axial CT contrast of the abdomen with IV contrast

A Segment I (caudate lobe) of the liver.
B Segment VI of the liver.
C Segment V of the liver.
D Hemiazygos vein.
E Azygos continuation of the inferior vena cava.

Couinaud was a French surgeon who divided the liver into eight functional segments, each with its own vascular and biliary drainage. (Figure 10.2). Bismuth further subdivided segment IV into IVA and IVB. The portal vein divides the liver into superior and inferior segments. The hepatic veins further subdivide these segments. The numbering of the segments can be remembered as they are numbered in approximate clockwise order, with segment II in the top left corner of the liver.

This image depicts an azygos continuation of the inferior vena cava. This anatomical variant occurs when the suprarenal inferior vena cava fails to form during embryological development. Associated situs anomalies are often present, but are not seen in this case.

See Question 8.19 for a further description of the liver segmental anatomy.

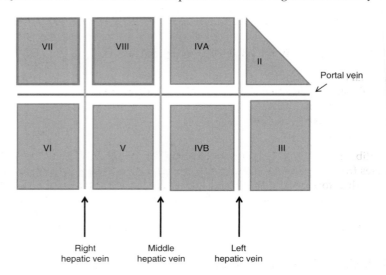

Figure 10.2 The segments of the liver

10.6 Coronal T1 MRI of the brachial plexus

A Right pectoralis minor muscle.
B Superior vena cava.
C Right sternocleidomastoid muscle.

D Left vertebral artery.
E Trunks of the left brachial plexus.

MRI is commonly used to assess the brachial plexus. The nerves are best demonstrated on T1-weighted imaging as they are surrounded in fat and appear hypo- or isointense to muscle. The brachial plexus is formed by the ventral rami of the nerve roots of C5–T1 and emerges between the scalenus medius and scalenus anterior muscles. The roots then merge to form three trunks:

Upper trunk	Formed by the roots C5/6
Middle trunk	Formed by the root C7
Lower trunk	Formed by the roots C8/T1

The trunks then cross the posterior triangle of the neck and form six divisions (three anterior and three posterior divisions), which pass posterior to the clavicle. The divisions then unite to form the three cords in the axilla:

Posterior cord	Formed by the posterior divisions of all three trunks
Lateral cord	Formed by the anterior divisions of the upper and middle trunks
Medial cord	Formed by the anterior division of the lower trunk

The cords then continue to form the nerves of the upper limb:

Posterior cord	Axillary nerve
	Radial nerve
Lateral cord	Musculocutaneous nerve
Medial cord	Ulnar nerve
Lateral and medial cord	Median nerve

10.7 Coronal T2 MRI of the right knee

A Iliotibial band.
B Lateral collateral ligament (or fibula collateral ligament).
C Popliteus tendon.
D Posterior cruciate ligament.
E Medial meniscus.

The iliotibial band is a longitudinal fibrous reinforcement of the fascia lata. It originates from the region of the anterior superior iliac spine and extends along the lateral thigh before attaching onto the lateral condyle of the tibia (Gerdy's tubercle). This band is crucial to the stability of the knee joint. In sport, the repeated rubbing of the iliotibial band against the lateral femoral epicondyle can cause inflammation and leads to iliotibial band syndrome, a common cause of lateral knee pain.

10.8 Axial CT of the abdomen with IV contrast

A Left external oblique muscle.
B Left latissimus dorsi muscle.
C Second part of the duodenum.
D Transverse colon.
E Retro-aortic left renal vein.

There are several common anatomical variants of the renal vasculature. This image depicts a retro-aortic left renal vein, which is seen in approximately 2–4% of the population. Although normally entirely asymptomatic, it can be implicated in 'posterior nutcracker syndrome', where the retro-aortic left renal vein is compressed between the aorta and the vertebrae leading to left renal venous hypertension. The symptoms of this include haematuria and flank pain.

The most common variant of the left renal venous system is the circumaortic renal vein (5–15% prevalence), in which the left renal vein bifurcates into a dorsal and ventral branch to encircle the aorta.

10.9 Sagittal T1 MRI of the right ankle

A Sinus tarsi.
B Navicular.
C Plantar aponeurosis.
D Calcaneum.
E Achilles tendon (calcaneal tendon).

The sinus tarsi is a cone-shaped anatomical space located in the lateral aspect of the foot between the inferolateral border of the talus and the superolateral border of the calcaneum. In healthy subjects the sinus tarsi is filled with fat, hence the high signal intensity seen on this T1-weighted image. It is an important area to review as sinus tarsi syndrome is a common cause of lateral hindfoot pain and instability.

The plantar aponeurosis is a strong fibrous fascial layer whose function is to stabilize the arch of the foot. It runs from the medial process of the calcaneal tuberosity to the heads of the metatarsal bones. The Achilles tendon is formed by the tendons of the soleus and gastrocnemius and inserts into the dorsal margin of the calcaneus. Rupture of the Achilles tendon typically occurs at the musculotendinous junction, located 2–6 cm above its insertion into the calcaneum.

10.10 Coronal cardiac CT

A Aortic valve.
B Right atrium.
C Left atrium.
D Papillary muscle of the left ventricle.
E Left ventricle wall/myocardium.

The aortic valve is found at the left ventricular outflow and separates the left ventricle from the ascending aorta. It is normally tricuspid, but in 1% of the population the valve is bicuspid. This is associated with early-onset aortic stenosis.

The papillary muscles lie within the ventricles of the heart. They attach to the cusps of the atrioventricular valves via the cordae tendinae, which can be seen as thin bands on CT. There are three in the right ventricle (anterior, posterior and septal) and two in the left ventricle (anterior and posterior). The muscles can rupture as a complication of myocardial infarction, which can result in valve prolapse.

10.11 Axial T1 MRI of the left elbow

A Common flexor tendon (medial epicondyle of the humerus).
B Ulnar nerve.
C Olecranon.
D Anconeus.
E Common extensor tendon (lateral epicondyle of the humerus).

The common flexor tendon is a common tendinous origin at the medial epicondyle of the humerus and is shared by a number of flexor muscles of the anterior compartment of the forearm. These muscles include the flexor carpi ulnaris and radialis, the palmaris longus and the pronator teres. The action of these muscles is to flex the wrist and elbow joints. Repetitive valgus stress to the elbow (such as in golf and baseball pitching) can cause microtrauma and inflammation of the flexor tendinous insertion, leading to medial epicondylitis, otherwise known as golfer's elbow.

The common extensor tendon is a common tendinous insertion at the lateral epicondyle of the humerus and is shared by a number of extensor muscles of the forearm. These muscles include the extensor carpi radialis, brevis and ulnaris, the extensor digitorum and the extensor digiti minimi. The action of these muscles is to extend the wrist and fingers. Repetitive wrist extension causes microtrauma and inflammation of the extensor tendinous insertion, leading to lateral epicondylitis, also known as tennis elbow.

The anconeus is a small muscle located at the posterior aspect of the elbow that takes its origin at the lateral epicondyle of the humerus and inserts into the olecranon of the ulna. It acts to extend the elbow and tighten the joint capsule.

The ulnar nerve is formed from the medial cord of the brachial plexus (C8–T1) and passes down the posterior aspect of the upper arm. It then courses through the cubital tunnel behind the medial epicondyle of the elbow before continuing through the anterior compartment of the forearm.

10.12 Coronal MRA of the kidneys

A Right renal capsule, right kidney.
B Right renal artery.
C Left lumbar artery.
D Left renal cortex.
E Left renal medulla.

The kidneys are encased by a tough fibrous capsule known as the renal capsule. The kidneys comprise an outer cortex and an inner medulla. The medulla contains the pyramids, named after their shape, and contains the functional unit of the kidney – the nephron. MRA of the renal arteries is commonly performed to assess for renal artery stenosis or in the assessment of a patient's vasculature prior to kidney donation.

10.13 X-ray of the left hand

A Left fifth proximal phalanx epiphysis.
B Left hamate.
C Left second metacarpal.
D Left capitate.
E Left distal radial epiphysis.

This child is 18 months old. The first metacarpal differs from the other four metacarpals in that its secondary ossification centre lies at the base and not at the head. These secondary ossification centres are generally all visible by age 2.

Ossification of the carpal bones occurs in a predictable sequence:

Bone	Average age at ossification
Capitate	2–4 months
Hamate	3–6 months
Triquetral	2–3 years
Lunate	4–5 years
Trapezium	6 years

Trapezoid	6–7 years
Scaphoid	6–7 years
Pisiform	11–12 years

10.14 Coronal STIR MRI of the prostate

A Bladder.
B Peripheral zone of the prostate.
C Central gland of the prostate.
D Left ischial tuberosity.
E Left hip capsule.

The prostate lies inferior to the bladder and encases the prostate urethra and ejaculatory ducts. It is cone-shaped, consisting of an apex (the tip of the cone, which sits on the urogenital diaphragm) and a base (which is situated along the inferior surface of the bladder). The prostate consists of three glandular zones:

Transition zone	Narrow area that surrounds the proximal urethra at the level of the ejaculatory ducts
	It is hypertrophy of this zone that is responsible for benign prostatic hypertrophy
Central zone	Surrounds the urethra above the level of the ejaculatory ducts
Peripheral zone	Subcapsular peripheral portion of the prostate that surrounds the distal urethra
	Largest part of the prostate accounting for 70% of the gland
	Roughly 80% of prostate cancers originate in this zone

MRI is the primary modality for the staging of prostate cancer as it is able to differentiate between disease confined to the prostate (T2 disease) and extra-prostatic disease (T3 disease). It is unable to differentiate between the transition and central zones of the prostate and is thus termed the central gland.

10.15 Axial T2 MRI of the breasts

A Right pectoralis major muscle.
B Right pectoralis minor muscle.
C Right breast fibroglandular tissue.
D Sternum.
E Left axillary lymph node.

Breast MRI is performed with the breasts placed within a surface coil and the patient lying prone. On T2-weighted imaging, mammary fat is seen as high-signal intensity, and the central fibroglandular tissue is seen as low signal intensity (as demonstrated here).

About 95% of the lymphatic drainage of the breast is to the axillary chain with the remaining 5% draining to the internal mammary chain. The axillary nodes are divided into three levels according to their relationship to the pectoralis minor muscle:

Level I nodes	Lateral to pectoralis minor
Level II nodes	Posterior to pectoralis minor
Level III nodes	Medial to pectoralis minor

10.16 Coronal T1 MRI of the right wrist

A Tendon of flexor digitorum profundus.
B pisiform.
C lunate.
D trapezium.
E Tendon of flexor pollicis longus.

Within the carpal tunnel, the tendons of the flexor digitorum profundus (FDP) and flexor pollicis longus (FPL) run in the same plane and deep to the tendons of the flexor digitorum superficialis (FDS). This image is at the level of the carpal bones and therefore must be at the level of the flexor digitorum profundus.

For more information on the carpal tunnel and the tendons of the flexor digitorum profundus and flexor digitorum superficialis, see Questions 5.20 and 9.7.

10.17 Axial CT of the chest

A Right middle lobe.
B Right horizontal (transverse) fissure.
C Right oblique fissure.
D Right lower lobe.
E Lingula of the left upper lobe.

The right lung is composed of three lobes – upper, middle and lower. The left lung is composed of two lobes – upper and lower, with an additional lingula lobe corresponding to the middle lobe of the right lung. Both lungs have an oblique fissure that extends from the spinous process of T2 posteriorly to the sixth costal cartilage anteriorly and separates all three lobes in the right lung and both lobes in the left lung. The transverse fissure is only located within the right lung and runs in line with the fourth costal cartilage to the meet the oblique fissure at the level of the sixth rib in the mid axillary line. It separates the right upper lobe from the right middle lobe.

See Question 7.6 for a further description of the lung fissures.

10.18 Selective angiogram of the inferior mesenteric artery

A Left colic artery.
B Marginal artery of Drummond.
C Inferior mesenteric artery.
D Sigmoid artery.
E Superior rectal artery.

The inferior mesenteric artery (IMA) is an anterior branch of the abdominal aorta, arising at the level of L3. It supplies the colon from the distal two-thirds of the transverse colon to the upper rectum. There are three major branches of the inferior mesenteric artery:

Left colic artery	Supplies the distal transverse colon and the descending colon
Sigmoid artery	Supplies the lower part of the descending colon and the sigmoid colon
Superior rectal artery	Supplies the upper rectum

The marginal artery of Drummond is a continuous arterial circle formed by anastomoses of the branches of the colic arteries of both the inferior and superior mesenteric arteries. It runs along the inner border of the colon.

10.19 AP X-ray of the left ankle

A Left talar dome.
B Left talonavicular joint.
C Left navicular.
D Left medial cuneiform.
E Left os subfibulare.

An os subfibulare is an accessory ossicle located just inferior the tip of the fibial epiphysis.

Other accessory ossicles around the ankle include:

Os tibiale externum	Also called an accessory navicular or os naviculare secundarium
	Ossicle located adjacent to the medial side of the navicular and within the tendon of the tibialis posterior
Os trigonum	Located posterior to the talus
Os supratalare	Located anterior superior to the talus
Os talotibiale	Located anterior to the tibia

For more information on the accessory ossicles of the foot see Question 1.20.

10.20 Angiogram of the pulmonary arteries

A Right ventricle.
B Pulmonary trunk.
C Left interlobar pulmonary artery.
D Left main pulmonary artery.
E Truncus anterior.

The venous catheter on this image is following the path of the left subclavian vein, brachiocephalic vein and superior vena cava. The inferior vena cava and the superior vena cava drain deoxygenated blood into the right atrium. Blood subsequently travels into the right ventricle via the tricuspid valve before entering the pulmonary trunk via the pulmonary valve. The pulmonary trunk originates from the right ventricle and divides into the right and left main pulmonary arteries under the aortic arch. The right main pulmonary artery then bifurcates into the truncus anterior (main branch to the upper lobe) and the interlobar artery (main branch to the middle and lower lobe). The slightly superior course of the left main pulmonary artery compared with the right explains why the left hilum is higher than the right in the 97% of individuals. It divides into two branches at the hilum – the upper division and the interlobar artery.

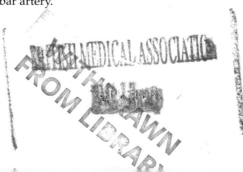